Blood Transfusion Therapy: A Physician's Handbook

Tenth Edition

2011

Draft 2 — 8/16/11

To purchase books or to inquire about other book services, including digital downloads and large-quantity sales, please contact our sales department:

- 866.222.2498 (within the United States)
- +1 301.215.6499 (outside the United States)
- +1 301.951.7150 (fax)
- www.aabb.org>Resources>Marketplace

AABB customer service representatives are available by telephone from 8:30 am to 5:00 pm ET, Monday through Friday, excluding holidays.

Editor
Karen E. King, MD

Contributing Editors
Nicholas Bandarenko, MD
Sally A. Campbell-Lee, MD
Laura W. Cooling, MD, MSc
Melissa M. Cushing, MD
Kenneth D. Friedman, MD
Gregory Pomper, MD

Handbook Series Editor
Jerome L. Gottschall, MD

AABB
8101 Glenbrook Road
Bethesda, Maryland 20814-2749

ISBN 978-1-56395-320-0
Printed in the United States

Contents

Preface

First published in 1983, *Blood Transfusion Therapy: a Physician's Handbook* is now in its 10th edition. Despite the many advances in transfusion medicine, the goal of the handbook remains the same—to present the most current principles of transfusion practice in a readily accessible handbook format. This 10th edition has been updated to be in compliance with the 27th edition of the AABB *Standards for Blood Banks and Transfusion Services*. Although still containing seven chapters, the entire handbook has been extensively reviewed and revised to include the latest recommendations on transfusion medicine practice based on the most up-to-date scientific information.

The Blood Components chapter includes information on all available blood products, including two recently approved platelet products—pooled leukocyte-reduced whole-blood-derived platelets that are screened for bacteria before release from the blood supplier and apheresis platelets suspended in a platelet additive solution (PAS). Chapter 2 on Plasma Derivatives includes descriptions and details related to all available plasma derivatives. In addition, the chapter has been updated with expanded information on prothrombin complex concentrates. The third chapter, Transfusion Practices, was extensively reorganized and rewritten to improve readability and accessibility of information. This chapter also includes an updated section on massive transfusion protocols.

Chapter 4 on Hemostatic Disorders contains expanded content on anticoagulant drugs with the latest information on oral direct-acting coagulation inhibitors. This chapter is organized and written to optimize clarity of an often confusing area of transfusion medicine. The chapter on Adverse Effects of Transfusion has been updated and has a new section on biovigilance. Chapter 6 on Hematopoietic Cellular Therapy includes expanded and updated information on hematopoietic growth factors and their appropriate use. The final chapter in the handbook is on therapeutic apheresis; this chapter has been extensively revised to reflect the 2010 ASFA guidelines regarding the indications for therapeutic apheresis.

Despite these many revisions and updates, the goal of this handbook continues to be simple: provide a thorough, yet convenient and concise resource that professionals turn to first. References have been updated to include the latest literature, facilitating access to more in-depth information, if needed.

The editors would like to thank the many individuals who contributed to this handbook. We gratefully acknowledge the diligence and hard work of the Contributing Editors, who were selected based on both their broad experience in transfusion medicine and their focused expertise in a particular area. Each Contributing Editor not only performed an intensive revision of the chapter in their area of expertise, but also reviewed the book as a whole. Their expertise and thoroughness are evident in the quality of this handbook. We would also like to thank the many dedicated members of the AABB staff who participated in this handbook. Our special thanks to Laurie Munk and Jennifer Boyer for their patience and assistance; without their help and support, this revision would not have been possible.

Karen E. King, MD
Jerome L. Gottschall, MD
Editors

BLOOD COMPONENTS

Concept of Blood Component Therapy

Blood component therapy refers to the transfusion of the specific part of blood that the patient needs, as opposed to the routine transfusion of Whole Blood. Because one donated unit can benefit several patients, this procedure not only conserves blood resources but also provides the optimal method of transfusing patients who require large amounts of a specific blood component. A unit of Whole Blood can be processed through a series of centrifugation steps into units of Red Blood Cells (RBCs), Platelets, and plasma or Cryoprecipitated Antihemophilic Factor (AHF) (see Table 1).

The plasma can also be used to manufacture several blood derivatives (eg, concentrates of coagulation factors, immune globulin, and plasma volume expanders), which are then treated to reduce or eliminate the risk of virus transmission. Apheresis technology can also be used to collect red cells, plasma, and/or platelets. Enough platelets for a single transfusion can be obtained by processing blood from a single donor by apheresis, thereby limiting the risk of disease transmission. Apheresis technology is also capable of collecting 2 RBC units or other combinations of components from a single donor. Thus, the availability of blood components and derivatives permits patients to receive specific hemotherapy that is more effective and usually safer than the use of Whole Blood.

Table 1. Blood Components and Plasma Derivatives

Component/Product	Composition	Volume	Indications
Whole Blood	RBCs (approx. Hct 40%); plasma; WBCs; platelets	500 mL	Increase both red cell mass and plasma volume (WBCs and platelets not functional; plasma deficient in labile clotting Factors V and VIII)
Red Blood Cells	RBCs (approx. Hct 75%); reduced plasma, WBCs, and platelets	250 mL	Increase red cell mass in symptomatic anemia (WBCs and platelets not functional)
Apheresis RBCs	RBCs (approx. Hct 55%)	300-350 mL	Increase red cell mass in symptomatic anemia
Red Blood Cells, Adenine-Saline Added	RBCs (approx. Hct 60%); reduced plasma, WBCs, and platelets; 100 mL of additive solution	330 mL	Increase red cell mass in symptomatic anemia (WBCs and platelets not functional)
RBCs Leukocytes Reduced (prepared by filtration)	>85% original volume of RBCs; $<5 \times 10^6$ WBCs; few platelets; minimal plasma	225 mL	Increase red cell mass; $<5 \times 10^6$ WBCs to decrease the likelihood of febrile reactions, immunization to leukocytes (HLA antigens) or CMV transmission
Washed RBCs	RBCs (approx. Hct 75%); $<5 \times 10^8$ WBCs; no plasma	180 mL	Increase red cell mass; reduce risk of allergic reactions to plasma proteins

Frozen RBCs; De-glycerolized RBCs	RBCs (approx. Hct 75%); <5 × 10^8 WBCs; no platelets; no plasma	180 mL	Increase red cell mass; minimize febrile or allergic transfusion reactions; use for prolonged RBC blood storage
Platelets	Platelets (>5.5 × 10^10/unit); RBCs; WBCs; plasma	50 mL	Bleeding due to thrombocytopenia or thrombocytopathy
Apheresis Platelets	Platelets (>3 × 10^11/unit); RBCs; WBCs; plasma	300 mL	Same as Platelets; sometimes HLA matched
Platelets Leukocytes Reduced	Platelets (as above); <5 × 10^6 WBCs per final dose of pooled Platelets	300 mL	Same as Platelets; <5 × 10^6 WBCs to decrease the likelihood of febrile reactions, alloimmunization to leukocytes (HLA antigens), or CMV transmission
Apheresis Platelets, Leukocytes Reduced	Platelets (>3 × 10^11/unit); <5 × 10^6 WBCs/unit; plasma	300 mL	Same as Apheresis Platelets; <5 × 10^6 WBCs to decrease the likelihood of febrile reactions, immunization to leukocytes (HLA antigens), or CMV transmission
FFP; FP24; Thawed Plasma	FFP and FP24: all coagulation factors Thawed Plasma: reduced Factors V and VIII	220 mL	Treatment of some coagulation disorders
Apheresis Granulocytes	Granulocytes (>1.0 × 10^10 PMN/unit); lymphocytes; platelets (>2.0 × 10^11/unit); some RBCs	220 mL	Provide granulocytes for selected patients with sepsis and severe neutropenia (<500 PMN/μL)

(Continued)

Table 1. Blood Components and Plasma Derivatives (Continued)

Component/Product	Composition	Volume	Indications
Cryoprecipitated AHF	Fibrinogen; Factors VIII and XIII; von Willebrand factor	15 mL	Deficiency of fibrinogen; Factor XIII; second choice in treatment of hemophilia A, von Willebrand disease; topical fibrin sealant
Factor VIII (concentrates; recombinant, human Factor VIII)	Factor VIII; trace amount of other plasma proteins (products vary in purity)	25 mL	Hemophilia A (Factor VIII deficiency); von Willebrand disease (selected products only)
Factor IX (concentrates, recombinant, human Factor IX)	Factor IX; trace amount of other plasma proteins (products vary in purity)	25 mL	Hemophilia B (Factor IX deficiency)
Albumin/PPF	Albumin, some α-, β-globulins	(5%); (25%)	Volume expansion
Immune Globulin	IgG antibodies; preparations for IV and/or IM use	Varies	Treatment of hypo- or agammaglobulinemia; disease prophylaxis; autoimmune thrombocytopenia (IV only)
Rh Immune Globulin	IgG anti-D; preparations for IV and/or IM use	1 mL	Prevention of hemolytic disease of the newborn due to D antigen; treatment of idiopathic thrombocytopenia (selected products only)
Antithrombin (concentrate; recombinant)	Antithrombin; trace amount of other plasma proteins	10 mL	Treatment of antithrombin deficiency

Product	Contents	Volume	Indications
Factor VIIa (recombinant)	Factor VIIa	1.0 mL (1.0 mg); 2.0 mL (2.0 mg); 5.0 mL (5.0 mg); 8.0 mL (8.0 mg)	Bleeding or prophylaxis before surgery for hemophilia A or B with inhibitors; Factor VII deficiency
Prothrombin Complex Concentrates (PCCs)	Factors IX, II, X and trace amount of Factor VII	25 mL	Hemophilia B (Factor IX deficiency) (Off-label use for warfarin reversal has been reported)
Fibrinogen concentrate	Fibrinogen	50 mL	Acute bleeding episodes for congenital fibrinogen deficiency
Factor XIII concentrate	Factor XIII	20 mL	Routine prophylaxis for congenital Factor XIII deficiency
Protein C concentrate	Protein C	5 mL; 10 mL	Prevention and treatment of venous thrombosis and purpura fulminans in patients with severe congenital protein C deficiency
Activated Prothrombin Complex Concentrates (aPCCs)	Factors II, IX, X (non-activated) and Factor VII (activated)	20 mL; 50 mL	Bleeding or prophylaxis before surgery for hemophilia A or B with inhibitors

RBCs = Red Blood Cells; Hct = hematocrit; WBCs = white cells; CMV = cytomegalovirus; PMN = polymorphonuclear leukocytes; FFP = Fresh Frozen Plasma; FP24 = Plasma Frozen Within 24 Hours After Phlebotomy; PPF = plasma protein fraction; IV = intravenous; IM = intramuscular.

During manufacture, the entire blood bag and any integrally attached satellite bags and needles are sterilized. Because the entire blood collection system is sterile, disposable, and never reused, the risk of donation is similar to that of any other phlebotomy. The blood collection set (including some apheresis systems) is considered a closed system, being open only at the tip of the needle used for donor phlebotomy. When the administration ports of a blood bag have been opened, however, the unit is considered an open system. Components prepared in an open system must be transfused within 24 hours if stored at 1 to 6 C; if stored at 20 to 24 C, components should be transfused within 4 hours to avoid possible bacterial contamination.[1(pp48-55)] To prepare components that have the maximal permitted shelf life, integral satellite bags should be used to ensure maintenance of the closed system. Alternatively, sterile connection devices are available; these devices permit sterile attachment of separate plastic bags.

Whole Blood

Description of Component

A unit of Whole Blood contains approximately 500 mL of blood and 70 mL of anticoagulant-preservative. The hematocrit of a typical unit is 36% to 44%. Whole Blood is stored in a monitored refrigerator at 1 to 6 C. The shelf life of Whole Blood depends on the preservative used in the blood collection bag [the shelf life of blood in citrate-phosphate-dextrose (CPD) is 21 days, and that of blood collected in CPD-adenine (CPDA-1) is 35 days]. See Table 2.

The level of 2,3-diphosphoglycerate (2,3-DPG), an intracytoplasmic molecule that facilitates the release of oxygen from hemoglobin, decreases during storage and is regenerated after infusion of the blood.[2] Whole Blood stored longer than 24 hours contains few viable platelets or granulocytes. In addition, levels

Table 2. Characteristics of Whole Blood Stored for 35 Days in CPDA-1 (n = 10)*

	Storage Time (Days)					
	0	7	14	21	35
Plasma dextrose (mg/dL)	432.00	374.00	357.00	324.00	282.00
Plasma sodium (mEq/L)	169.00	162.00	159.00	157.00	153.00
Plasma potassium (mEq/L)	3.30	12.30	17.60	21.70	17.20
Plasma chloride (mEq/L)	84.00	81.00	79.00	77.00	79.00
Plasma bicarbonate (mEq/L)	12.00	17.00	12.50	12.20	8.00
Whole-blood pH	7.16	6.94	6.93	6.87	6.73
Whole-blood lactate (mg/dL)	19.00	62.00	91.00	130.00	202.00
Plasma LDH (units)	296.00	1002.00	1222.00	1457.00	1816.00

(Continued)

Table 2. Characteristics of Whole Blood Stored for 35 Days in CPDA-1 (n = 10)*
(Continued)

	0	7	14	21	35
Whole-blood ammonia (mg/dL)	82.00	280.00	423.00	521.00	703.00
Plasma hemoglobin (mg/dL)	0.50	13.10	24.70	24.70	45.60
WBCs (10^3/µL)	7.20	4.00	3.00	2.80	2.40
Hematocrit (%)	35.00	36.00	35.00	36.00	36.00
RBC hemoglobin (g/dL)	12.00	12.00	12.00	12.00	12.00
RBCs (10^6/µL)	4.00	4.00	3.90	3.90	3.90
RBC 2,3-DPG (mmol/g Hb)[†]	13.20	—	—	—	0.70
RBC ATP (mmol/g Hb)	4.18	—	—	—	2.40

*Latham JT, Bove JR, Weirich FL. Chemical and hematologic changes in stored CPDA-1 blood. Transfusion 1982;22:158-9.
[†]Moore GL, Peck CC, Sohmer PR, Zuck TF. Some properties of blood stored in anticoagulant CPDA-1 solution. Transfusion 1981;21:135-7.
CPDA-1 = citrate-phosphate-dextrose-adenine; LDH = lactate dehydrogenase; WBCs = white cells; RBCs = Red Blood Cells; DPG = diphosphoglycerate; ATP = adenosine triphosphate; Hb = hemoglobin.

of Factor V and Factor VIII decrease with storage. Levels of stable clotting factors, however, are well-maintained in units of Whole Blood during storage. See Table 3.

Indications

Whole Blood provides both oxygen-carrying capacity and blood volume expansion. The primary indication is for treating patients who are actively bleeding and who also have sustained a loss of more than 25% of their total blood volume. These patients are at risk of developing hemorrhagic shock. The use of Whole Blood in massively bleeding patients (those who receive one blood volume, or more than 10 RBC units, in less than 24 hours) may limit donor exposures, if RBCs and plasma would otherwise be given (see Urgent and Massive Transfusion in Chapter 3). Unless a patient needs volume replacement in addition to oxygen-carrying capacity, the use of Whole Blood may result in circulatory overload, especially if rapid infusion is attempted. If the patient is thrombocytopenic, platelets should be administered. Plasma should be given to replace needed labile clotting factors. There is limited justification for the use of "fresh" Whole Blood (ie, blood collected within the previous 48 hours) in infants undergoing certain complex cardiac surgical procedures.[3] Fresh Whole Blood has also been used by the military in the setting of massive transfusion for resuscitation following combat-related injuries.[4,5] Because of the limited indications for the use of Whole Blood and the more efficient use of selected blood components, Whole Blood is generally not available.

Contraindications and Precautions

Whole Blood may result in circulatory overload, especially if rapidly infused. Whole Blood should not be given to patients with chronic anemia who are normovolemic and who require only an increase in red cell mass; RBCs should be used in such patients to decrease the risk of transfusion-associated circulatory overload. See Chapter 5: Adverse Effects of Blood Transfusion.

Table 3. In-Vitro Properties of Blood Clotting Factors

Factor	Plasma Concentration Required for Hemostasis*	Half-Life of Transfused Factor	Recovery in Blood (as % of Amount Transfused)	Stability in Liquid Plasma and Whole Blood (4 C Storage)
I (fibrinogen)	100-150 mg/dL	3-6 days	50%	Stable
II	40 U/dL (40%)	2-5 days	40-80%	Stable
V	10-25 U/dL (15-25%)	15-36 hours	80%	Unstable[†]
VII	5-20 U/dL (5-10%)	2-7 hours	70-80%	Stable
VIII	10-40 U/dL (10-40%)	8-12 hours	60-80%	Unstable[‡]
IX	10-40%	18-24 hours	40-50%	Stable
X	10-20%	1.5-2 days	50%	Stable

XI	15-30%	3-4 days	90-100%	Stable
XII	—	—	—	Stable
XIII	1-5%	6-10 days	5-100%	Stable
vWF	25-50%	3-5 hours	—	Unstable

*Upper limit usually refers to surgical hemostasis.
†50% remains at 14 days.
‡25% remains at 24 hours.

Adapted from Colman RW. Hemostasis and thrombosis: Basic principles and clinical practice. 3rd ed. Philadelphia: Lippincott, 1993:958, and Rizza ER. Management of patients with inherited blood coagulation defects. In: Bloom AL, Thomas DP, eds. Haemostasis and thrombosis. London: Churchill Livingstone, 1981:371.

Dose and Administration

In an adult, 1 unit of Whole Blood will increase the hemoglobin level by about 1 g/dL or the hematocrit by about 3% to 4%. In pediatric patients, a Whole Blood transfusion of 8 mL/kg will result in an increase in hemoglobin of approximately 1 g/dL. Whole Blood must be administered through a blood administration set containing a 170- to 260-micron filter. The rate of infusion depends on the clinical condition of the patient, but each unit or aliquot should be infused within 4 hours.

Red Blood Cells

Description of Component

RBCs are prepared from Whole Blood by the removal of 200 to 250 mL of plasma. RBC components are also collected through apheresis technology. The use of apheresis devices enables collection of RBCs and a second blood component or a 2-unit RBC collection. The indications, contraindications, precautions, dosage, and administration of RBC components obtained by apheresis are the same as those for RBC components obtained from whole blood donation. RBC units are stored at 1 to 6 C in one of several anticoagulant-preservative solutions. These solutions contain various amounts and/or types of preservative agents (eg, buffer, dextrose, adenine, and mannitol). The resultant RBC components have different hematocrits and shelf lives. RBCs stored in additive solutions (AS) have hematocrits of 55% to 65% and a shelf life of 42 days, whereas RBCs stored in CPDA-1 have hematocrits of 65% to 80% and a shelf life of 35 days.[2,6,7] RBCs stored in CPD have hematocrits similar to those of RBCs stored in CPDA-1 but have a shelf life of only 21 days. RBCs are not a source of functional platelets or granulocytes. RBCs and

Whole Blood have the same oxygen-carrying capacity because they contain the same number of red cells.

Indications

RBCs are indicated for treatment of anemia in normovolemic patients who require an increase in oxygen-carrying capacity and red cell mass. The transfusion requirements of each patient should be based on clinical status rather than on any predetermined hematocrit or hemoglobin value.[8]

Contraindications and Precautions

Risks associated with RBC infusion are the same as those encountered with Whole Blood. See Chapter 5: Adverse Effects of Blood Transfusion.

Dose and Administration

In an adult with an average blood volume, 1 RBC unit will increase the hemoglobin level by about 1 g/dL or the hematocrit by about 3%. In a pediatric patient, an RBC transfusion of 10 to 15 mL/kg will raise the hemoglobin level by 2 to 3 g/dL or the hematocrit by about 6%. RBCs must be transfused through a blood administration filter (170 to 260 microns). The higher hematocrit of CPD or CPDA-1 RBCs results in greater viscosity, which may slow the transfusion rate. To decrease viscosity, 50 to 100 mL of isotonic sodium chloride (0.9% USP) may be used to dilute the RBCs in CPD or CPDA-1, but this practice must be balanced against the risk of hypervolemia. The lower hematocrit of AS RBC units permits more rapid infusion rates. For patients at risk for circulatory overload and for pediatric patients, concern over the additional volume resulting from the 100 mL of AS may warrant concentrating the component by centrifugation or sedimentation. Other than isotonic saline, no solutions or medications should be added to RBCs or infused through the same tubing, unless approved for this use by the Food and Drug Administration (FDA)[1(p42)] (see Administration of Blood in Chapter 3).

Red Blood Cells Leukocytes Reduced

Description of Component

RBC units contain 1 to 3×10^9 leukocytes.[9,10] AABB *Standards for Blood Banks and Transfusion Services* specifies that leukocyte-reduced RBCs must contain $<5 \times 10^6$ leukocytes/unit while retaining 85% of the original red cells.[1(p26)] The standard 170-micron blood filter does not remove leukocytes.

Leukocyte reduction is best achieved by filtration of the unit in the blood center shortly after blood collection (prestorage filtration) or in the transfusion service laboratory before blood issue (laboratory filtration). Leukocyte reduction may be performed at the time of transfusion by passing the blood through one of several commercially available bedside blood filters. Prestorage and laboratory filtration have several advantages over bedside filtration of RBCs. These methods are generally more effective than bedside filtration, as they more consistently leave $<10^6$ leukocytes/unit. Additionally, prestorage and laboratory filtration can provide an immediately available inventory of Red Blood Cells Leukocytes Reduced with a normal shelf life, permitting quality control of residual leukocyte content.[11,12] Prestorage leukocyte reduction is the optimal method of leukocyte reduction because it also results in lower levels of cytokine generation in blood bags during storage and results in a lower risk of febrile nonhemolytic transfusion reactions.[13-17] Some apheresis technologies are able to produce RBCs Leukocytes Reduced that have the same advantages as prestorage leukocyte-reduced products. Bedside filtration usually leaves $<5 \times 10^6$ leukocytes in the transfused blood[18]; however, the success of this method depends on the duration of unit storage, the initial leukocyte content of the unit, and the proper use of the filter. Some bedside leukocyte reduction filters have been associated with hypotension and other adverse effects. Because of quality-control issues, bedside filtration is not the preferred method of leukocyte reduction.

Indications

Red Blood Cells Leukocytes Reduced are indicated for use in patients who have had repeated febrile reactions in association with the transfusion of RBCs or Platelets and as prophylaxis against alloimmunization for patients in whom intensive or long-term hemotherapy is anticipated.[12] Patients who have received frequent transfusions and females who have had multiple pregnancies may become alloimmunized to leukocyte antigens. Alloimmunization can be manifested as febrile transfusion reactions and/or as refractoriness to platelet transfusion (see Platelets section). Studies indicate that allogeneic leukocytes are responsible for the development of alloimmunization to HLA antigens[19] and that antibodies to leukocyte antigens are responsible for many recurrent febrile transfusion reactions.[20]

The routine prophylactic use of leukocyte-reduced blood components diminishes the likelihood of primary alloimmunization to leukocyte antigens.[12,21] Patients who have a high likelihood of becoming alloimmunized (eg, patients with chronic transfusion requirements) may be considered candidates for the prophylactic use of leukocyte-reduced blood components.[12,21] A decision to use leukocyte-reduced RBCs prophylactically in an effort to prevent alloimmunization should be made before the first blood transfusion. The decision implies a commitment to use leukocyte-reduced Platelets as well as RBCs (see Platelets Leukocytes Reduced section).

Certain immunosuppressed, cytomegalovirus (CMV)-seronegative patients such as allogeneic hematopoietic progenitor cell transplant recipients are susceptible to severe transfusion-transmitted CMV disease.[22] Although some controversy does exist,[23] clinical studies of such patients indicate that leukocyte-reduced blood components are as effective in preventing transmission of CMV infection as are blood components obtained from CMV-seronegative donors.[24-26] Even with the use of universal leukocyte reduction, transfusion-transmitted CMV may still occur.[27] Transfusion of cellular blood components is associated with immunomodulation—that is, changes in host immune function. This property was once employed to prolong the survival of renal allografts, but it has been supplanted by improved immunosuppressive drug therapy. Most, but not all, prospective randomized studies have shown that the use of leukocyte-reduced blood lowers the incidence of wound infection in selected surgical patients. However, the mechanism of this effect is unclear, and the use of leukocyte-reduced blood components for this purpose is controversial.[28,29]

Although required in several countries, universal leukocyte reduction of cellular blood components has been implemented voluntarily by many blood centers in the United States.

Contraindications and Precautions

Patients who receive RBCs Leukocytes Reduced are subject to the same volume-related hazards as are those who receive RBCs. Red Blood Cells Leukocytes Reduced may contain 5% to 10% fewer red cells as a result of loss in the filters. This component is not indicated to prevent transfusion-associated graft-vs-host disease (TA-GVHD), because cases of TA-GVHD have been reported after its use. At this time, only irradiation is approved for the prevention of TA-GVHD.

Dose and Administration

RBC units that have undergone leukocyte reduction by prestorage filtration or laboratory filtration must be transfused through a blood administration filter. However, administration of RBCs through a bedside leukocyte reduction filter eliminates the need for the standard blood filter. Personnel who administer blood through bedside leukocyte reduction filters should be thoroughly familiar with the requirements for their use in order to achieve optimal leukocyte reduction, provide acceptable blood flow rates, and ensure against excessive loss of red cells.

Washed Red Blood Cells

Description of Component

RBC units may be washed with 1 to 2 L of sterile normal saline by use of specially designed machines. The washed red cells are suspended in sterile saline, usually at hematocrits of 70% to 80%, with a volume of approximately 180 mL. Saline washing removes all but traces of plasma, reduces the concentration of leukocytes, and removes platelets and cellular debris. Saline washing may be performed at any time during the shelf life of a unit of blood, but because washing is ordinarily performed in an open system, the resultant component can be stored for only 24 hours at 1 to 6 C.

Indications

The predominant indication for Washed RBCs in adults is to prevent recurrent or severe allergic reactions. In IgA-deficient or haptoglobin-deficient patients at risk for anaphylaxis, Washed RBCs can prevent life-threatening reactions. Washed RBCs should be considered for the prevention of transfusion-associated hyperkalemia in high-risk patients. Washed RBCs should not be used when RBCs Leukocytes Reduced are indicated.

Contraindications and Precautions

Because of the risk of bacterial contamination, Washed RBCs may be stored at 1 to 6 C for no longer than 24 hours after preparation.[1(p50)] Washing is associated with the loss of 10% to 20% of the red cells. Transfusion hazards associated with washed cells are similar to those associated with RBCs. Washed RBCs are capable of transmitting hepatitis[30] and other infectious diseases. Because they contain sufficient numbers of viable leukocytes, this component will not prevent TA-GVHD.

Dose and Administration

All units must be infused through a blood administration set containing a 170- to 260-micron filter. Because a unit of Washed RBCs provides a smaller red cell mass than does a unit of RBCs, patients who are chronically transfused with Washed RBCs may require additional transfusions to achieve the desired hematocrit.

Frozen Red Blood Cells; Deglycerolized Red Blood Cells

Description of Component

Frozen RBCs are prepared by adding glycerol, a cryoprotective agent, to blood that is usually less than 6 days old. RBC units may be rejuvenated and then frozen up to 3 days after expiration. The unit is frozen at –65 or –200 C (depending on the concentration of cryoprotective agent) for as long as 10 years. Once thawed, the unit is washed to remove the glycerol by use of a series of saline-glucose solutions. The unit is then reconstituted in sterile saline, usually at a hematocrit of 70% to 80%. The final product must contain at least 80% of the original red cell volume. The thawing and deglycerolization process results in a delay between the time of order and when the unit is available. When prepared in an open system, this component may be stored at 1 to 6 C for no longer than 24 hours.[1(p49)] When prepared in a closed system, the unit may be stored at 1 to 6 C for 14 days.

Indications

This technique is useful for long-term preservation of RBC units of a rare phenotype and autologous RBCs. Because the process of deglycerolization requires extensive washing, this product can be used for patients with a history of severe allergic reactions, including patients with IgA deficiency. For leukocyte reduction alone, the use of deglycerolized RBCs is not indicated.

Contraindications and Precautions

RBCs that have been frozen and deglycerolized carry the same risks and hazards as do Washed RBCs. This component is capable of transmitting infectious diseases and has been shown to contain viable lymphocytes.[31]

Dose and Administration

All units must be administered through a blood administration set with a 170- to 260-micron filter. Deglycerolized RBCs provide a smaller red cell mass because of the loss of red cells during processing. Therefore, patients transfused with these units could require additional transfusions to achieve a desired hematocrit.

Platelets

PLATELETS

Description of Component

Platelets, prepared from individual units of Whole Blood by centrifugation, have been referred to as random-donor platelets or whole-blood-derived platelet concentrates. Although units should contain at least 5.5×10^{10} platelets, most units contain more than this amount. One collection center reports an average yield of 9.08×10^{10} platelets per unit.[32] Platelets should be suspended in sufficient plasma (usually 50 to 70 mL) to maintain a pH greater than 6.2 throughout the storage period.[1(p28)] Platelets, which may be stored in the blood bank for as long as 5 days at 20 to 24 C with constant gentle agitation, have nearly normal posttransfusion recovery and survival.[33] They are typically pooled at the time of issue; Platelets pooled in an open system expire 4 hours from the time the system is opened.

Indications

Platelets are indicated for treatment of bleeding associated with thrombocytopenia (platelet counts usually <50,000/μL) or for use in patients with functionally abnormal platelets (congenital or acquired).[34-36] They are also indicated during surgery or before certain invasive procedures in patients who have platelet counts <50,000/μL. Prophylactic transfusion of Platelets may be indicated for patients who have platelet counts <5,000 to 10,000/μL associated with marrow hypoplasia resulting from chemotherapy, tumor invasion, or primary aplasia.[37-39] This range may be higher for patients with complicating clinical factors.[38] Additionally, platelet transfusions are often included in massive transfusion protocols. In the setting of massive bleeding, improved survival has been seen in patients who receive a higher ratio of platelet to red cell transfusions.[40,41]

Contraindications and Precautions

In patients with rapid platelet destruction, such as idiopathic (immune) thrombocytopenia (ITP) and disseminated intravascular coagulation (DIC), transfusion solely to achieve a platelet increment is not clinically appropriate. In such patients, platelet transfusion should be used only in the presence of active bleeding with clinical monitoring. Platelet transfusions are relatively contraindicated in patients with thrombotic thrombocytopenic purpura (TTP) and heparin-induced thrombocytopenia (HIT); platelets are indicated only if these patients are bleeding.[42] Patients with thrombocytopenia caused by septicemia or hypersplenism may also fail to demonstrate an increment in platelet count.

Transfusion reactions, including febrile nonhemolytic and allergic reactions, may occur. Fever should not be treated with antipyretics containing aspirin (acetylsalicylic acid), because aspirin will inhibit platelet function. Repeated transfusions may lead to alloimmunization to HLA and other antigens and may result in the development of a "refractory" state manifested by unresponsiveness to platelet transfusion (see Management of Platelet Alloimmunization in Chapter 3). Some transfusion reactions appear to be associated with the accumulation of cytokines in stored platelets, which suggests that the reactions may be prevented by prestorage leukocyte reduction of platelets.[43,44]

Platelets may contain up to 0.5 mL of red cells per unit, with as much as 2 to 4 mL per pooled product. Because of the potential presence of this small amount of red cells in a platelet transfusion, patients who are D-negative generally should receive platelets only from a D-negative donor. If D-positive Platelets must be transfused to D-negative females of childbearing potential or to children, prevention of D immunization by the use of Rh Immune Globulin should be considered.

Platelets containing ABO-incompatible plasma may be transfused; for example, this may occur when ABO-compatible platelets are not available or when HLA-matched platelets are required. Plasma contained in transfused units of ABO-incompatible Platelets may cause a positive direct antiglobulin test (DAT) result and, very rarely, hemolysis in the recipient.[45,46] Whenever possible, ABO-plasma-compatible Platelets should be selected. Other approaches include volume reduction, instituting maximum volume limitations per 24 hours, and screening of donors to identify high-titer ABO antibodies; there is currently no standard, broadly accepted approach.[47,48]

Rapid infusion may cause circulatory overload and other complications related to increased intravascular volume. The risks of transfusion-transmitted infectious diseases are similar to those associated with RBCs, and, because platelets from multiple donors must be pooled to obtain an adequate dose for an adult, those risks are multiplied.

Bacterial contamination of Platelets is of special concern because this component is stored at room temperature.[49] Required prevention strategies, including drawline diversion pouches and implementation of methods to detect bacterial contamination before products are issued, are not 100% effective and posttransfusion sepsis remains a concern.[50,51]

Dose and Administration

The usual dose for a thrombocytopenic bleeding patient is 1 unit of Platelets per 10 kg body weight (typically, 4 to 8 units for an adult). A recent multi-center trial investigated the optimal platelet dose for patients undergoing hematopoietic stem cell transplantation or chemotherapy and receiving prophylactic platelet transfusions for the prevention of bleeding; the specific dose of platelets (between 1.1×10^{11} to 4.4×10^{11} platelets per square meter of body surface area) did not affect the incidence of bleeding.[52] Patients receiving the lower dose did require an increased number of transfusions.

One unit of Platelets usually increases the platelet count in a 70-kg adult by 5000/µL. Repeated failure to achieve hemostasis or the expected increment in platelet count may signify the refractory state.[34,53] Immune refractoriness to platelets is most commonly associated with antibodies to HLA antigens and rarely with those to platelet-specific antigens. Clinical refractoriness to platelets is associated with bleeding, amphotericin, splenomegaly, DIC, fever, sepsis, viremia, drugs, veno-occlusive disease, or hematopoietic progenitor cell transplantation.[54] Refractoriness is often suspected on the basis of repeatedly poor clinical response to platelet transfusion and a poor posttransfusion platelet count increment. The corrected count increment (CCI) may be calculated more accurately as follows:

$$CCI = \frac{(\text{Post-tx plt ct}) - (\text{pre-tx plt ct}) \times BSA \times 10^{11}}{\text{Number of Platelets transfused}}$$

where Post-tx plt ct = posttransfusion platelet count, Pre-tx plt ct = pretransfusion platelet count, and BSA = body surface area in square meters. Each unit of Platelets contains a minimum of 5.5 $\times 10^{10}$ platelets, and a unit of Apheresis Platelets contains at least 3×10^{11} platelets.

A CCI of >7500 to 10,000 from a sample drawn 10 minutes to 1 hour after transfusion or a CCI of >4500 from a sample drawn

18 to 24 hours after transfusion is considered acceptable (ie, not indicative of refractoriness).[55,56] Patients who repeatedly have poor clinical or 1-hour CCI responses are more likely to be immune refractory to platelet transfusion and to pose difficult management problems (see Management of Platelet Alloimmunization in Chapter 3). Patients who are refractory because of the emergence of HLA or platelet alloantibodies usually require HLA-matched, HLA-selected, or crossmatched platelets.[53] Patients who have adequate 1-hour CCI responses, but poor 24-hour CCI recovery, are most likely refractory because of nonimmune causes and may require more frequent or larger doses of platelets.

Platelets must be administered through a blood administration set with a 170- to 260-micron filter. Testing of platelets for red cell compatibility is not necessary, unless 2 mL or more of red cells are present. Because platelets express ABO antigens, it may be preferable to give platelets from donors who are ABO compatible with the patient's plasma in order to optimize recovery. Likewise, it is preferable to give donor plasma that is compatible with the recipient's red cells, especially if large amounts are given to recipients with small blood volumes.[45] Platelet units may be pooled before administration or infused individually. Platelets may be volume reduced to prevent circulatory overload or to diminish the transfusion of ABO-incompatible plasma. Platelets should be transfused within 4 hours after pooling. Gamma-irradiated platelets must be selected for patients at risk for TA-GVHD.

APHERESIS PLATELETS

Description of Component

Apheresis Platelets are collected from an individual donor during a 1- to 2-hour cytapheresis procedure, and must contain at least 3×10^{11} platelets.[1(p28)] This number is equal to 4 to 6 units of Platelets. The volume of plasma in the component varies from 200 to 400 mL. The number of leukocytes and red cells varies with the apheresis technique. Apheresis Platelets collected by using recently developed technologies may be considered leukocyte reduced when quality is controlled under current good manufacturing practice regulations.

Indications

Apheresis Platelets are indicated in the same clinical settings as Platelets. In order to limit donor exposures, Apheresis Platelets may be used in patients who are not refractory.[57] Apheresis Platelets that are either HLA-matched, HLA-selected, or crossmatch-compatible with the recipient are indicated for patients who are unresponsive to whole-blood-derived Platelets because of HLA alloimmunization. Physicians treating patients who are refractory to Platelets should consult with the transfusion service medical director to determine the best therapeutic alternatives (see Management of Platelet Alloimmunization in Chapter 3).

Contraindications and Precautions

Adverse effects and hazards are similar to those for Platelets. Acute hemolytic transfusion reactions have been reported with the transfusion of Apheresis Platelets containing ABO-incompatible plasma.[58]

Dose and Administration

One unit of Apheresis Platelets will usually increase the platelet count of a 70-kg adult by 30,000 to 60,000/μL. Compatibility testing is the same as for Platelets. If the Apheresis Platelets were collected by a technique that allowed the product to contain 2 mL or more of red cells, red cell compatibility testing must be performed. Preferably, the donor plasma should be ABO-compatible with the recipient's red cells, if the product is not group-specific. Administration is similar to that for Platelets.

PLATELETS LEUKOCYTES REDUCED

Description of Component

Platelets contain leukocytes (approximately 0.5 to 1×10^8/unit of Platelets), which are not removed by the standard 170-micron blood filter.[59-61] Platelets Leukocytes Reduced should contain $<8.3 \times 10^5$ leukocytes per unit[1(p28)] and, when pooled, a final dose of less than 5×10^6 leukocytes.[1(p28)] The number of leukocytes remaining in the component after leukocyte reduction varies with the type of platelet component, the number of units processed, and the type of leukocyte reduction procedure employed. The passage of platelets through leukocyte reduction filters generally removes 99.9% of leukocytes and less than 10% of the platelets in the platelet component.[60,61]

The FDA has recently approved a system to produce a pooled platelet product that is leukocyte reduced, screened for bacteria, and may be stored for up to 5 days. These products provide an available pooled platelet inventory that meets the requirements of bacterial screening.[62]

Indications

See the earlier discussion of RBCs Leukocytes Reduced. Platelets Leukocytes Reduced are indicated as prophylaxis against HLA alloimmunization in selected patients who are destined to receive long-term transfusion therapy.[21,63,64] The decision to use Platelets Leukocytes Reduced in an effort to prevent alloimmunization should optimally be made before the first blood transfusion. This decision implies a commitment to use RBCs Leukocytes Reduced to ensure that all cellular components are leukocyte reduced. Platelets Leukocytes Reduced are also effective in reducing the risk of CMV transmission.[24]

Contraindications and Precautions

Although the use of Platelets Leukocytes Reduced may eliminate febrile reactions in patients who are already alloimmunized to HLA antigens, their use will not improve the low platelet recovery rate or short platelet survival time. Obtaining a good platelet increment in such patients nearly always requires the use of HLA-matched, HLA-selected, or crossmatched platelets.[63] Clinical studies show that various reactions (eg, chills) are associated with transfusion of platelets that have been stored for several days.[43,44,65] Evidence suggests that such reactions may be caused by the infusion of cytokines, including interleukins (eg, IL-1, IL-6, and IL-8), and of tumor necrosis factor-alpha (TNF-α), which have been generated by leukocytes during storage.[65-67] There is no evidence to suggest that these reactions can be prevented by bedside filtration; however, clinical data have shown that prestorage leukocyte reduction can decrease the incidence of such reactions.[15,16] Other hazards are similar to those of Platelets that have not undergone leukocyte reduction.

Dose and Administration

Personnel who prepare Platelets Leukocytes Reduced or administer platelets through leukocyte reduction filters should be thoroughly familiar with the requirements for their use, which vary from one filter to another. Leukocyte reduction filters are manufactured to be component-specific, and care must be taken to ensure that an appropriate filter has been selected for use. The use of a leukocyte reduction filter in the administration set when platelets are transfused at the bedside eliminates the need for any other blood administration filter.

APHERESIS PLATELETS LEUKOCYTES REDUCED

The majority of cytapheresis instruments available in the United States are reliably capable of reducing the leukocyte content of Apheresis Platelets to $<5 \times 10^6$/unit.[68,69] Apheresis Platelets Leukocytes Reduced do not appear to have an advantage over pooled Platelets Leukocytes Reduced in reducing the frequency of alloimmunization and refractoriness in patients requiring long-term transfusion support.[21] See Platelets Leukocytes Reduced.

The FDA has approved a platelet additive solution (PAS) for use in a leukocyte-reduced apheresis platelet system. The final product contains approximately 65% PAS and 35% residual plasma, and it may be stored for up to 5 days at 20 to 24 C. Although CCIs related to these products have been variable, clinical bleeding outcomes have been comparable to conventional platelets stored in plasma and these products meet FDA criteria for pH, recovery, and survival at 5 days.[70] These products offer several potential advantages, including decreased risk of transfusion-related adverse events such as hemolysis due to ABO-incompatibility, allergic transfusion reactions and transfusion-related acute lung injury (TRALI).

Apheresis Granulocytes

Description of Component

Granulocytes are usually prepared by cytapheresis of a single donor. They may also be prepared as a "buffy coat" preparation from single units of fresh blood for neonatal granulocyte transfusion.[71] Each unit contains $\geq 1.0 \times 10^{10}$ granulocytes and various amounts of lymphocytes, platelets, and red cells; the unit is then suspended in 200 to 300 mL of plasma. Hydroxyethyl starch (HES, a red-cell-sedimenting agent) is used in the collection. Corticosteroids are routinely administered to the donor to facilitate granulocyte collection. Although not used at all centers, administration of granulocyte colony-stimulating factor (G-CSF) to healthy donors can significantly increase the collection of granulocytes to 4 to 8×10^{10} granulocytes/bag.[72,73] Healthy donors who receive G-CSF at doses of 5 to 10 μg/kg may experience side effects such as bone pain, myalgia, arthralgia, nausea/vomiting, or headaches.[72,74] These symptoms generally require no treatment or can be treated successfully with acetaminophen.[74] Fluid retention has been observed in some donors who receive repeated daily doses of corticosteroids and G-CSF. Long-term follow-up of volunteer granulocyte donors suggests that G-

CSF/dexamethasone stimulation appears to be safe.[75] Granulocytes collected from G-CSF-stimulated donors appear to function normally, although they differ phenotypically from granulocytes collected from unstimulated donors with increased expression of adhesion molecules.[72] Transfusion of G-CSF-mobilized granulocyte components typically results in measurable increases in peripheral blood granulocyte counts of 1000/μL or more, which are sustained above baseline for 1 to 2 days.[76] The presence of platelets in granulocyte concentrates is often beneficial because many neutropenic patients are also thrombocytopenic.[76] Granulocytes should be transfused as soon as possible, but they may be stored at 20 to 24 C for up to 24 hours after collection.[77,78]

Indications

The decision to use granulocytes should be made in consultation with the transfusion service physician. The patient typically has neutropenia (neutrophil count <500/μL), infection (preferably documented) for 24 to 48 hours, lack of responsiveness to appropriate antibiotics or other modes of therapy, marrow showing myeloid hypoplasia, and a reasonable chance for recovery of marrow function. Granulocyte transfusions may also be beneficial for neonatal patients with sepsis[79] and patients with hereditary neutrophil function defects, including chronic granulomatous disease. Randomized studies have suggested that granulocyte transfusions of at least 1×10^{10} per transfusion could be beneficial in selected neutropenic patients.[80-83] It has been suggested that clinical response to granulocyte transfusion therapy may be limited by the dose of granulocytes administered, and it is possible that the larger doses obtained with G-CSF-stimulated donors may lead to enhanced therapeutic benefit. Randomized clinical studies with G-CSF-enhanced doses of granulocytes are needed to define the clinical indications and efficacy of this therapy.[81] Currently, a Phase III randomized, controlled trial sponsored by the National Institutes of Health [the Resolving Infections in Neutropenia with Granulocytes (RING) Study] is under way to evaluate the efficacy of G-CSF/dexamethasone-mobilized granulocyte transfusions in neutropenic patients who have received chemotherapy and have probable or proven infections.[82]

Contraindications and Precautions

Successful treatment of the infected neutropenic patient includes appropriate antimicrobial therapy and/or the use of hematopoietic growth factors, in addition to possible use of granulocyte transfusions. If recovery of marrow function is doubtful, granulocyte transfusions are unlikely to alter the ultimate clinical course of a neutropenic patient. Patients alloimmunized to HLA may be less likely to benefit from whole-blood-derived granulocytes.[84] Chills, fever, and allergic reactions may occur and are minimized by slow infusion rates, diphenhydramine and/or meperidine, steroids, and/or nonaspirin antipyretics. In some patients, severe febrile and pulmonary reactions to Apheresis Granulocytes (eg, when infused in conjunction with amphotericin) may preclude their further use.[85] There is a risk of viral disease transmission, especially CMV; consequently, CMV-seronegative patients who are at high risk for CMV disease, such as patients undergoing allogeneic progenitor cell transplants, should receive CMV-seronegative granulocytes. Immunization to HLA and red cell antigens may occur as well.[86] In most clinical circumstances, gamma irradiation should be performed to prevent TA-GVHD. Gamma irradiation in doses used to prevent TA-GVHD does not impair the function of granulocytes. The use of leukocyte reduction filters is contraindicated for granulocytes.

Dose and Administration

Although most blood centers do not perform HLA typing on Apheresis Granulocytes, red cell compatibility testing must be performed because of the large number of red cells present. Although single daily granulocyte transfusions are often given, the kinetics of transfused granulocytes from G-CSF-stimulated donors may allow for every-other-day transfusion.[76] A blood administration set with a 170- to 260-micron filter must be used; leukocyte reduction filters should not be used.

Plasma Components

Description of Component

Several plasma alternatives can be used for coagulation factor replacement, including Fresh Frozen Plasma (FFP), Plasma Frozen Within 24 Hours After Phlebotomy (FP24), and Thawed Plasma. FFP is prepared from Whole Blood by separating and freezing the plasma at less than or equal to –18 C within 8 hours of phlebotomy, if collected in CPD, CP2D, or CPDA-1. FFP may also be obtained by using apheresis procedures. Apheresis technology allows for the collection of the equivalent of 2 units of plasma during a single donation. FP24 is prepared from Whole Blood by separating and freezing the plasma at less than or equal to –18 C within 24 hours of phlebotomy. Except for Factor VIII, FP24 contains similar levels of coagulation factors and inhibitors as FFP. Despite a variable reduction in Factor VIII, the Factor VIII levels in FP24 are generally within the normal range of human plasma.[87] Plasma may be stored for as long as 1 year at –18 C or colder. The volume of a typical unit is 200 to 250 mL. Under these conditions, the loss of Factors V and VIII, the labile clotting factors, is minimal. One mL of FFP contains approximately 1 unit of coagulation factor activity. Thawed Plasma is thawed FFP or FP24 stored for up to 4 days beyond the outdate of the plasma. The volume is also 200 to 250 mL. The levels of Factor VIII and Factor V decline during storage, although the latter does not fall below the hemostatic level of 35%.[88] Studies have shown that Thawed Plasma prepared from FFP and from FP24 have comparable levels of coagulation activities.[89,90] Solvent/detergent-treated plasma, a pooled plasma product that has been treated with a solvent and a detergent to eliminate lipid-enveloped viruses, is used in Europe but is no longer available in the United States.[91]

Indications

Plasma is indicated for use in bleeding patients or patients undergoing an invasive procedure with multiple coagulation factor deficiencies (eg, those secondary to liver disease, DIC, and the dilutional coagulopathy resulting from massive blood or volume replacement).[35,92,93] The latter is a common indication for plasma transfusion; however, the level of coagulopathy requiring replacement is controversial.[35,92,93] Plasma transfusion is indicated for the rapid reversal of warfarin effect in a bleeding patient or in the setting of emergency surgery; an alternative approach includes the use of prothrombin complex concentrates (see Chapter 2: Plasma Derivatives). Because minor prolongations in coagulation tests are not predictive of excessive bleeding, the prothrombin time (PT) or activated partial thromboplastin time (aPTT) should be indicative of factor levels of 30% or lower, or the international normalized ratio (INR) should be 2.0 or higher before prophylactic plasma is used (Table 3).[35,92,94,95] Plasma is indicated in patients with congenital factor deficiencies for which there is no coagulation concentrate available, such as deficiencies of Factor II, V, X, or XI. Plasma may also be used as primary therapy and as the principal replacement solution in therapeutic plasma exchange procedures for the treatment of TTP and atypical hemolytic uremic syndrome. Plasma Cryoprecipitate Reduced has also been employed in refractory cases of TTP.[96]

Contraindications and Precautions

Plasma should not be used to provide blood volume expansion, because it exposes patients unnecessarily to the risk of transfusion-transmitted diseases. Albumin, plasma protein fraction (PPF), or other colloid or crystalloid solutions that do not transmit infection are safer components to use for blood volume expansion. Similarly, plasma should not be used as a source of protein in nutritionally deficient patients. In general, plasma has a risk of infectious disease transmission equal to that of Whole Blood. Certain viruses [eg, CMV and human T-cell lymphotropic virus, type I (HTLV-I)] do not appear to be transmitted by plasma because they are associated exclusively with leukocytes.[97] Allergic reactions can occur with plasma infusion.[98] IgA-deficient patients at risk for anaphylaxis should receive IgA-deficient plasma. Plasma products have been associated with TRALI, prompting strategies to reduce this risk (See Chapter 5: Adverse Effects of Transfusion).[99]

Dose and Administration

The dose of plasma depends on the clinical situation and the underlying disease process. When plasma is given for coagulation factor replacement, the dose is 10 to 20 mL/kg (3 to 6 units in an adult). This dose would be expected to increase the level of coagulation factors by 20% immediately after infusion. Plasma is one of the components given to patients with vitamin K deficiency when it is not possible to wait for the administered vitamin K to take effect. Posttransfusion assessment of the patient's coagulation status is important, and monitoring of coagulation function with clinical assessment, PT, aPTT, or specific factor assays is critical. As with all blood components, plasma must be given through a filter. Plasma thawed at 30 to 37 C should be transfused as soon as possible, but it must be transfused within 24 hours; it can be stored for up to 5 days as Thawed Plasma. After thawing, FFP, FP24, and Thawed Plasma should be stored at 1 to 6 C. Compatibility testing is not required, but ABO-compatible plasma must be used.

Cryoprecipitated Antihemophilic Factor

Description of Component

Cryoprecipitated AHF is a concentrated source of certain plasma proteins. It is prepared by thawing 1 unit of FFP at 1 to 6 C. After it is thawed, the supernatant plasma is removed, which leaves the cold-precipitated protein plus 10 to 15 mL of plasma in the bag. This material is then refrozen at –18 C or colder within 1 hour and has a shelf life of 1 year. Cryoprecipitated AHF contains concentrated Factor VIII:C (the procoagulant activity), Factor VIII:VWF (von Willebrand factor), fibrinogen, and Factor XIII. Each bag of Cryoprecipitated AHF contains approximately 80 to 120 units of Factor VIII, at least 150 mg of fibrinogen,[1(p27)] and about 20% to 30% of the Factor XIII present in the initial unit. Approximately 40% to 70% of the VWF present in the initial unit of FFP is recovered in the cryoprecipitate. Cryoprecipitated AHF is the main source of concentrated fibrinogen for the treatment of patients with acquired deficiency.

Indications

Cryoprecipitated AHF may be indicated for the treatment of congenital or acquired fibrinogen deficiency or Factor XIII deficiency. Although the FDA recently approved a plasma-derived fibrinogen concentrate product for the treatment of bleeding in patients with congenital fibrinogen deficiency, many institutions may not be routinely maintaining the product in inventory.[100] Cryoprecipitate is not indicated in hemophilia A and von Willebrand disease when factor concentrates are available. Because it does not contain clinically significant amounts of other coagulation factors, Cryoprecipitated AHF is not indicated as the sole treatment for DIC, but it is an important component in the treatment of disorders with low fibrinogen. Cryoprecipitated AHF has also been reported to be beneficial in treating the bleeding tendency associated with uremia[101]; however, its use should be restricted to those who are unresponsive to nontransfusion therapy (eg, dialysis or desmopressin), because the latter approach is free of the potential infectious complications of Cryoprecipitated AHF.[102] The use of Cryoprecipitated AHF as a fibrin sealant has been largely replaced by the use of commercially available products (eg, Tisseel, Baxter Healthcare, Glendale, CA).[103] See Chapter 2: Plasma Derivatives.

Contraindications and Precautions

Cryoprecipitated AHF should not be used to treat patients with deficiencies of factors other than fibrinogen or Factor XIII. It should be used as second-line therapy for hemophilia A and von Willebrand disease. ABO-compatible cryoprecipitate is not required, because of the small amount of plasma, although this volume of plasma may be clinically significant in infants. In rare instances, infusion of large numbers of ABO-incompatible units of Cryoprecipitated AHF can cause hemolysis; a positive DAT can be seen with infusion of smaller doses. The risk of infectious disease transmission, for each unit of Cryoprecipitated AHF given, is the same as that for FFP.

Dose and Administration

Before infusion, the cryoprecipitate is thawed at 30 to 37 C. Each unit will increase fibrinogen by 5 to 10 mg/dL in an average-size adult. In a bleeding patient, a reasonable target level for fibrinogen is 100 mg/dL. Cryoprecipitated AHF is administered through a blood administration set with a 170- to 260-micron filter; no compatibility test is required. If a single unit of Cryoprecipitated AHF is thawed but not used immediately, it may be stored no more than 6 hours at room temperature. Once pooled, Cryoprecipitated AHF must be transfused within 4 hours after pooling, regardless of whether it is prepared in an open or closed system.

Oxygen Therapeutics

Oxygen therapeutics (red cell substitutes) are not clinically available in the United States at this time.

Pathogen Reduction

The risk of transmission of various pathogens via blood transfusion continues to decrease as a result of improvements in donor screening and laboratory testing. Concern remains over the transmission of viruses in the "window period" of infection, the transmission of organisms for which routine testing is not available, and the transmission of an infectious agent before it has been identified. Because of these limitations, recent efforts have focused on developing technologies that treat blood components to eliminate contaminating pathogens without the need to specifically test for their presence. Currently, the addition of a solvent and detergent to eliminate enveloped viruses is licensed by the FDA in the manufacturing of plasma derivatives.[104] Solvent/detergent-treated plasma is no longer available in the United States. Photoactivated psoralens[105] are being investigated for use in cellular and plasma components. S-303, PEN110, and riboflavin are novel compounds for pathogen reduction of red cell components. These compounds all interfere with DNA and RNA replication.[106] Although available in Europe, these pathogen inactivation and/or pathogen reduction technologies are not currently approved for use in the United States.[107]

References

1. Carson TH, ed. Standards for blood banks and transfusion services. 27th ed. Bethesda, MD: AABB, 2011.
2. Moore GL, Ledford ME, Peck CC. The in vitro evaluation of modifications in CPD-adenine anticoagulated-preserved blood at various hematocrits. Transfusion 1980;20: 419-26.

3. Mou SS, Giroir BP, Molitor-Kirsch EA, et al. Fresh whole blood versus reconstituted blood for pump priming in heart surgery in infants. N Engl J Med 2004;351:1635-44.

4. Perkins JG, Cap AP, Spinella PC, et al. Comparison of platelet transfusion as fresh whole blood versus apheresis platelets for massively transfused combat trauma patients. Transfusion 2011;51:242-52.

5. Hakre S, Peel SA, O'Connell RJ, et al. Transfusion-transmissible viral infections among US military recipients of whole blood and platelets during Operation Enduring Freedom and Operation Iraqi Freedom. Transfusion 2011;51: 473-85.

6. Heaton A, Miripol J, Aster R, et al. Use of Adsol preservation solution for prolonged storage of low viscosity AS-1 red blood cells. Br J Haematol 1984;57:467-78.

7. Simon TL, Marcus CS, Myhre BA, Nelson EJ. Effects of AS-3 nutrient-additive solution on 42 and 49 days of storage of red cells. Transfusion 1987;27:178-82.

8. Klein HG, Spahn DR, Carson JL. Red blood cell transfusion in clinical practice. Lancet 2007;370:415-26.

9. Meryman HT, Hornblower M. The preparation of red cells depleted of leukocytes. Transfusion 1986;26:101-6.

10. Sirchia G, Rebulla P, Parravicini A, et al. Leukocyte depletion of red cell units at the bedside by transfusion through a new filter. Transfusion 1987;27:402-5.

11. Pietersz RN, Steneker I, Reesink HW. Prestorage leukocyte depletion of blood products in a closed system. Transfus Med Rev 1993;7:17-24.

12. Lane TA, Anderson KC, Goodnough LT, et al. Leukocyte reduction in blood component therapy. Ann Intern Med 1992;117:151-62.

13. Stack G, Snyder EL. Cytokine generation in stored platelet concentrates. Transfusion 1994;34:20-5.

14. Stack G, Baril L, Napychank P, Snyder EL. Cytokine generation in stored, white-cell-reduced, and bacterially contaminated units of red cells. Transfusion 1995;35:199-203.

15. Yazer MH, Podlosky L, Clarke G, Nahirniak SM. The effect of prestorage WBC reduction on the rates of febrile nonhemolytic transfusion reactions to platelet concentrates and RBC. Transfusion 2004;44:10-15.

16. Paglino JC, Pomper GJ, Fisch GS, et al. Reduction of febrile but not allergic reactions to RBCs and platelets after conversion to universal prestorage leukoreduction. Transfusion 2004;44:16-24.

17. King KE, Shirey RS, Thoman SK, et al. Universal leukoreduction decreases the incidence of febrile nonhemolytic transfusion reactions to RBCs. Transfusion 2004;44:25-9.

18. Rebulla P, Porretti L, Bertolini F, et al. White cell-reduced red cells prepared by filtration: A critical evaluation of current filters and methods for counting residual white cells. Transfusion 1993;33:128-33.

19. Claas FHJ, Smeenk RJT, Schmidt R, et al. Alloimmunization against the MHC antigens after platelet transfusions is due to contaminating leukocytes in the platelet suspension. Exp Hematol 1981;9:84-9.

20. Perkins HA, Payne R, Ferguson J, Wood M. Nonhemolytic febrile transfusion reactions. Quantitative effects of blood components with emphasis on isoantigenic incompatibility of leukocytes. Vox Sang 1966;11:578-99.

21. TRAP Study Group. Leukocyte reduction and ultraviolet B irradiation of platelets to prevent alloimmunization and refractoriness to platelet transfusions. N Engl J Med 1997; 337:1861-9.

22. Sayers MH, Anderson KC, Goodnough LT, et al. Reducing the risk for transfusion-transmitted cytomegalovirus infection. Ann Intern Med 1992;116:55-62.

23. Nichols WG, Price TH, Gooley T, et al. Transfusion-transmitted cytomegalovirus infection after receipt of leukoreduced blood products. Blood 2003;101:4195-200.

24. Bowden RA, Cays MJ, Schoch G, et al. Comparison of filtered blood (FB) to seronegative blood products (SB) for prevention of cytomegalovirus (CMV) infection after marrow transplant. Blood 1995;86:3598-603.

25. Narvios AB, Przepiorka D, Tarrand J, et al. Transfusion support using filtered unscreened blood products for cytomegalovirus-negative allogeneic marrow transplant recipients. Bone Marrow Transplant 1998;22:575-7.
26. Laupacis A, Brown J, Costello B, et al. Prevention of post-transfusion CMV in the era of universal WBC reduction: A consensus statement. Transfusion 2001;41:560-9.
27. Wu Y, Zou S, Cable R, et al. Direct assessment of cytomegalovirus transfusion-transmitted risks after universal leukoreduction. Transfusion 2010;50:776-86.
28. Blajchman MA. Allogeneic blood transfusions, immunomodulation, and postoperative bacterial infection: Do we have the answers yet? (editorial) Transfusion 1997;37:121-5.
29. Blajchman MA, Dzik WH, Vamvakas EC, et al. Clinical and molecular basis of transfusion-induced immunomodulation: Summary of the proceedings of a state-of-the-art conference. Transfus Med Rev 2001;15:108-35.
30. Haugen RK. Hepatitis after the transfusion of frozen red cells and washed red cells. N Engl J Med 1979;301:393-5.
31. Chaplin H. Frozen red cells revisited. N Engl J Med 1984; 311:1696-8.
32. Hoeltge GA, Shah A, Miller JP. An optimized strategy for choosing the number of platelet concentrates to pool. Arch Pathol Lab Med 1999;123:928-30.
33. Schiffer CA, Lee EJ, Ness PM, Reilly J. Clinical evaluation of platelets stored for one to five days. Blood 1986;67: 1591-4.
34. NIH consensus development conference. Platelet transfusion therapy. JAMA 1987;257:1777-80.
35. College of American Pathologists. Practice parameter for the use of fresh-frozen plasma, cryoprecipitate, and platelets. JAMA 1994;271:777-81.
36. British Committee for Standards in Haematology, Blood Transfusion Task Force. Guidelines for the use of platelet transfusions. Br J Haematol 2003;122:10-23.

37. Gmur J, Burger J, Schanz U, et al. Safety of stringent prophylactic platelet transfusion policy for patients with acute leukaemia. Lancet 1991;338:1223-6.

38. Rebulla P, Finazzi G, Marangoni F, et al. The threshold for prophylactic platelet transfusions in adults with acute myeloid leukemia. N Engl J Med 1997;337:1870-5.

39. Heckman KD, Weiner GJ, Davis CS, et al. Randomized study of prophylactic platelet transfusion threshold during induction therapy for adult acute leukemia: 10,000/µL versus 20,000/µL. J Clin Oncol 1997;15:1143-9.

40. Dente CJ, Shaz BH, Nicholas JM, et al. Improvements in early mortality and coagulopathy are sustained better in patients with blunt trauma after institution of a massive transfusion protocol in a civilian level I trauma center. J Trauma 2009;66:1616-24.

41. Johansson PI, Stensballe J. Hemostatic resuscitation for massive bleeding: The paradigm of plasma and platelets—a review of the current literature. Transfusion 2010;50:701-10.

42. Warkentin TE, Greinacher A, Koster A, Lincoff AM. Treatment and prevention of heparin-induced thrombocytopenia: American College of Chest Physicians evidence-based clinical practice guidelines (8th ed). Chest 2008;133 (6 Suppl):340S-380S.

43. Muylle L, Joos M, Wouters E, et al. Increased tumor necrosis factor alpha (TNF-α), interleukin 1 (IL-1), and interleukin 6 (IL-6) levels in the plasma of stored platelet concentrates: Relationship between TNF-α and IL-6 levels and febrile transfusion reactions. Transfusion 1993;33: 195-9.

44. Heddle NM, Blajchman MA. The leukodepletion of cellular blood products in the prevention of HLA-alloimmunization and refractoriness to allogeneic platelet transfusions. Blood 1995;85:603-6.

45. Pierce RN, Reich LM, Mayer K. Hemolysis following platelet transfusions from ABO-incompatible donors. Transfusion 1985;25:60-2.

46. Herman JH, King KE. Apheresis platelet transfusions: Does ABO matter? Transfusion 2004;44:802-4.

47. Quillen K, Sheldon SL, Daniel-Johnson JA, et al. A practical strategy to reduce the risk of passive hemolysis by screening plateletpheresis donors for high-titer ABO antibodies. Transfusion 2011;51:92-6.

48. Cooling L. ABO and platelet transfusion therapy. Immunohematology 2007;23:20-33.

49. Blajchman MA, Goldman M. Bacterial contamination of platelet concentrates: Incidence, significance and prevention. Semin Hematol 2001;38(Suppl 11):20-6.

50. Eder AF, Kennedy JM, Dy BA, et al. Bacterial screening of apheresis platelets and the residual risk of septic transfusion reactions: The American Red Cross experience (2004-2006). Transfusion 2007;47:1134-42.

51. Fuller AK, Uglik KM, Savage WJ, et al. Bacterial culture reduces but does not eliminate the risk of septic transfusion reactions to single-donor platelets. Transfusion 2009;49:2588-93.

52. Slichter AJ, Kaufman RM, Assmann SF, et al. Dose of prophylactic platelet transfusions and prevention of hemorrhage. N Engl J Med 2010;362:600-13.

53. Yankee RA, Grumet FC, Rogentine GN. Platelet transfusion therapy: The selection of compatible platelet donors for refractory patients by lymphocyte HLA typing. N Engl J Med 1969;281:1208-12.

54. Bishop JF, McGrath K, Wolf MM, et al. Clinical factors influencing the efficacy of pooled platelet transfusions. Blood 1988;71:383-7.

55. Kickler TS, Braine HG, Ness PM, et al. A radiolabeled antiglobulin test for crossmatching platelet transfusions. Blood 1983;61:238-42.

56. Daly PA, Schiffer CA, Aisner J, Wiernik PH. Platelet transfusion therapy: One-hour posttransfusion increments are valuable in predicting the need for HLA-matched preparations. JAMA 1980;243:435-8.

57. Ness P, Braine H, King K, et al. Single-donor platelets reduce the risk of septic platelet transfusion reactions. Transfusion 2001;41:857-61.

58. Fung MK, Downes KA, Shulman IA. Transfusion of platelets containing ABO-incompatible plasma. A survey of 3156 North American Laboratories. Arch Pathol Lab Med 2007;131:909-16.

59. Menitove JE, McElligott MC, Aster RH. Febrile transfusion reaction: What blood component should be given next? Vox Sang 1982;42:318-21.

60. Sniecinski MR, O'Donnell B, Nowicki B, Hill LR. Prevention of refractoriness and HLA-alloimmunization using filtered blood products. Blood 1988;71:1402-7.

61. Andreu J, Dewailly C, Leberre MC, et al. Prevention of HLA immunization with leukocyte-poor packed red cells and platelet concentrates obtained by filtration. Blood 1988;72:964-9.

62. Vassallo RR, Wagner SJ, Einarson M, et al. Maintenance of in vitro properties of leukoreduced whole blood-derived pooled platelets after a 24-hour interruption of agitation. Transfusion 2009;49:2131-5.

63. Slichter SJ. Platelet transfusion therapy. Hematol Oncol Clin North Am 1990;4:291-311.

64. Seftel MD, Growe GH, Petraszko T, et al. Universal prestorage leukoreduction in Canada decreases platelet alloimmunization and refractoriness. Blood 2004;103:333-9.

65. Heddle NM, Klama L, Singer J, et al. The role of plasma in platelet concentrates in transfusion reactions. N Engl J Med 1994;331:625-8.

66. Aye MT, Palmer DS, Giulivi A, Hashemi S. Effect of filtration of platelet concentrates on the accumulation of cytokines and platelet release factors during storage. Transfusion 1995;35:117-24.

67. Ferrara JL. The febrile platelet transfusion reaction: A cytokine shower. Transfusion 1995;35:89-90.

68. Bertholf MF, Mintz PD. Comparison of plateletpheresis using two cell separators and identical donors. Transfusion 1989;29:521-3.

69. Anderson KC, Gorgone BC, Wahlers E, et al. Preparation and utilization of leukocyte poor apheresis platelets. Transfus Sci 1991;12:163-70.

70. Vassallo RR, Adamson JW, Gottschall JL, et al. In vitro and in vivo evaluation of apheresis platelets stored for 5 days in 65% platelet additive solution /35% plasma. Transfusion 2010;50:2376-85.

71. Strauss RG, Rohret PA, Randels MJ, Winegarden DC. Granulocyte collection. J Clin Apher 1991;6:241-3.

72. Dale DC, Liles WC, Llewellyn C, et al. Neutrophil transfusions: Kinetics and functions of neutrophils mobilized with granulocyte colony-stimulating factor and dexamethasone. Transfusion 1998;38:713-21.

73. Jendiroba DB, Lichtiger B, Anaissie E, et al. Evaluation and comparison of three mobilization methods for the collection of granulocytes. Transfusion 1998;38:722-8.

74. Stroncek DF, Clay ME, Petzoldt ML, et al. Treatment of normal individuals with granulocyte colony-stimulating factor: Donor experiences and the effects on peripheral blood CD34+ cell counts and on the collection of peripheral blood stem cells. Transfusion 1996;36:601-10.

75. Quillen K, Byrne P, Yau YY, Leitman SF. Ten-year follow-up of unrelated volunteer granulocyte donors who have received multiple cycles of granulocyte-colony-stimulating factor and dexamethasone. Transfusion 2009;49:513-18.

76. Adkins D, Spitzer G, Johnston M, et al. Transfusions of granulocyte colony-stimulating factor-mobilized granulocyte components to allogeneic transplant recipients: Analysis of kinetics and factors determining posttransfusion neutrophil and platelet counts. Transfusion 1997;37:737-48.

77. Lane TA. Granulocyte storage. Transfus Med Rev 1990; 4:23-34.

78. Lightfoot T, Leitman SF, Stroncek DF. Storage of G-CSF-mobilized granulocyte concentrates. Transfusion 2000;40:1104-10.

79. Cairo MS. The use of granulocyte transfusion in neonatal sepsis. Transfus Med Rev 1990;4:14-22.

80. Strauss RG, Connett JE, Gale RP, et al. A controlled trial of prophylactic granulocyte transfusions during initial induction chemotherapy for acute myelogenous leukemia. N Engl J Med 1981;305:597-603.

81. Strauss R. Neutrophil (granulocyte) transfusions in the new millennium (editorial). Transfusion 1998;38:710-2.

82. Dale DC, Price TH. Granulocyte transfusion therapy: A new era? Curr Opin Hematol 2009;16:1-2.

83. Vamvakas EC, Pineda AA. Meta-analysis of clinical studies of the efficacy of granulocytes transfusions in the treatment of bacterial sepsis. J Clin Apher 1996;11:1-9.

84. Price TH. Granulocyte transfusion: Current status. Semin Hematol 2007;44:15-23.

85. Dutcher JP, Kendall J, Norris D, et al. Granulocyte transfusion therapy and amphotericin B: Adverse reactions? Am J Hematol 1989;31:102-8.

86. Heim KF, Fleisher TA, Stroncek DF, et al. The relationship between alloimmunization and posttransfusion granulocyte survival: Experience in a chronic granulomatous disease cohort. Transfusion 2011;51:1154-62.

87. Eder AF, Sebok MA. Plasma components: FFP, FP24, and thawed plasma. Immunohematology 2007;23:150-7.

88. Downes KA, Wilson E, Yomtovian R, Sarode R. Serial measurement of clotting factors in thawed plasma stored for 5 days (letter). Transfusion 2001;41:570.

89. Yazer MH, Cortese-Hassett A, Triulzi DJ. Coagulation factor levels in plasma frozen within 24 hours of phlebotomy over 5 days of storage at 1 to 6 C. Transfusion 2008;48:2525-30.

90. Scott E, Puca K, Heraly J, et al. Evaluation and comparison of coagulation factor activity in fresh-frozen plasma and

24-hour plasma at thaw and after 120 hours of 1 to 6 C storage. Transfusion 2009;49:1584-91.

91. Hellstern P. Solvent/detergent-treated plasma: Composition, efficacy, and safety. Curr Opin Hematol 2004;11:346-50.

92. NIH consensus development conference. Fresh frozen plasma: Indications and risks. JAMA 1985;253:551-3.

93. O'Shaughnessy DF, Atterbury C, Bolton Maggs P, et al. British Committee for Standards in Haematology, Blood Transfusion Task Force. Guidelines for the use of fresh-frozen plasma, cryoprecipitate and cryosupernatant. Br J Haematol 2004;126:11-28.

94. American Society of Anesthesiologists Task Force on Perioperative Blood Transfusion and Adjuvant Therapies. Practice guidelines for perioperative blood transfusion and adjuvant therapies. Anesthesiology 2006;105:198-208.

95. Holland L, Sarode R. Should plasma be transfused prophylactically before invasive procedures? Curr Opin Hematol 2006;13:447-51.

96. Rock G, Shuman KH, Sutton DM, et al. Members of the Canadian Apheresis Group. Cryosupernatant as replacement fluid for plasma exchange in thrombotic thrombocytopenic purpura. Br J Haematol 1996;94:383-6.

97. Bowden R, Sayers M. The risk of transmitting cytomegalovirus infection by fresh-frozen plasma. Transfusion 1990;30:762-3.

98. Braunstein AH, Oberman HA. Transfusion of plasma components. Transfusion 1984;24:281-6.

99. Eder AF, Herron RM, Strupp A, et al. Effective reduction of transfusion-related acute lung injury risk with male-predominant plasma strategy in the American Red Cross (2006-2008). Transfusion 2010;50:1732-42.

100. Sorensen B, Bevan D. A critical evaluation of cryoprecipitate for replacement of fibrinogen. Br J Hematol 2010; 149:834-43.

101. Janson PA, Jubelirer SJ, Weinstein MJ, Deykin D. Treatment of the bleeding tendency in uremia with cryoprecipitate. N Engl J Med 1980;303:1318-22.

102. Remuzzi G. Bleeding in renal failure. Lancet 1988;i:1205-8.

103. Gibble JW, Ness PM. Fibrin glue: The perfect operative sealant? Transfusion 1990;30:741-7.

104. Klein HG, Dodd RY, Dzik WH, et al. Current status of solvent/detergent-treated frozen plasma. Transfusion 1998;38:102-7.

105. McCullough J, Vesole DH, Benjamin RJ, et al. Therapeutic efficacy and safety of platelets treated with a photochemical process for pathogen inactivation: The SPRINT Trial. Blood 2004;104:1534-41.

106. AuBuchon JP, Pickard CA, Herschel LH, et al. Production of pathogen-inactivated RBC concentrates using PEN110 chemistry: A phase I clinical study. Transfusion 2002;42:146-52.

107. Klein HG, Glynn SA, Ness PM, Blajchman MA. Research opportunities for pathogen reduction/inactivation of blood components: Summary of an NHLBI workshop. Transfusion 2009;49:1262-68.

Factor VIII Concentrates

Description of Products

Factor VIII preparations can be derived from human plasma or produced by recombinant technology.

Recombinant Factor VIII (rFVIII) is produced in established hamster cell lines. First-generation rFVIII contains animal- and/or human-plasma-derived proteins in the culture medium and in the final formulation vial. Second-generation rFVIII contains plasma proteins in the medium but not in the final formulation. Third-generation rFVIII does not contain any plasma-derived proteins in the culture medium or in the final formulation vial.

Because rFVIII is thought to be extraordinarily safe in regard to transmitting human infectious organisms, it has become the product of choice for treating patients with hemophilia A.[1,2] Controversy exists, however, with regard to a questionable higher risk of inhibitor development (antibodies directed against the coagulation factor) with recombinant products.[3,4] The higher cost of recombinant products can also play a role in product choice.

Human-plasma-derived Factor VIII concentrate [also referred to as antihemophilic factor (AHF)] is prepared by fractionation of pooled human plasma that is frozen soon after collection. Several types of human-plasma-derived Factor VIII concentrates are available. All products take the form of a sterile, stable, lyophilized concentrate, but differ in terms of protein purity. The purity is usually expressed by the specific activity, which refers to units of clotting factor per milligram of protein.

The purest human-derived products are produced through immunoaffinity chromatography that uses murine monoclonal antibodies to a portion of the Factor VIII complex.[5] The purity of these products is greater than 90% before the addition of albumin, which is used as a stabilizer. Several intermediate-purity Factor VIII concentrates that are produced in a manner that retains von Willebrand factor (VWF) are also on the market. Humate-P (CSL Behring, King of Prussia, PA) and Alphanate (Grifols Biologicals, Los Angeles, CA) are labeled in VWF ristocetin cofactor activity units and are indicated for the treatment of von Willebrand disease. In addition, a new VWF/FVIII high-purity concentrate replacement therapy developed specifically for von Willebrand disease (Wilate Octapharma, Hoboken, NJ) is now available.

Various procedures are used to inactivate viruses in Factor VIII products and reduce the risk of infectious disease transmission[6]; these procedures include a combination of pasteurization and solvent/detergent treatment and affinity chromatography preparation. It should be noted that no treatment procedure or combination of procedures completely eliminates the risk of virus transmission. This may be particularly relevant with respect to certain non-lipid-enveloped viruses (such as hepatitis A and parvovirus B19), as well as emerging pathogens. Several novel Factor VIII products designed to prolong half-life and decrease immunogenicity are under development. A half-life range of 8 to 12 hours has been reported for all currently available Factor VIII products. Active bleeding, surgery, or inhibitor development may reduce the half-life.

For indications and treatment, see Chapter 4: Hemostatic Disorders.

Factor IX and Prothrombin Complex Concentrates

Description of Products

Factor IX preparations are available from recombinant and plasma-derived sources.

Recombinant Factor IX concentrate is produced in a Chinese hamster ovary cell line. Because no human products are used, it is not thought to transmit human infectious diseases. For this reason, recombinant Factor IX is the treatment of choice for new patients with hemophilia B and for those with limited exposure to human-derived Factor IX products.[1,7]

Human plasma coagulation Factor IX is a highly purified preparation containing trace (nontherapeutic) amounts of Factors II, VII, and X. These concentrates were developed by advanced chromatographic methods or monoclonal antibody purification in order to provide a less thrombogenic material. Prothrombin complex concentrate (PCC) is a term that refers to crude preparations of Factor IX that contain other vitamin-K-dependent proteins to a varying extent, but are generally labeled by Factor IX content. Products approved in the United States include Bebulin VH (Baxter Healthcare, Deerfield, IL) and Profilnine SD (Grifols Biologicals, Los Angeles, CA). These products are referred to as three-factor concentrates and contain mainly Factors II, IX, and X and low amounts of Factor VII. In other countries, products that include therapeutic levels of Factor VII are available and are referred to as four-factor concentrates. Off-label use of PCCs in the treatment of Factor X deficiency has been reported.[8] Recently, the off-label use of PCCs in the urgent reversal of vitamin K anticoagulant effect has become increasingly common, but may need supplementation with a source of Factor VII.[9,10] Human-derived Factor IX concentrates are heat-treated and/or solvent/detergent-treated to decrease the risk of infectious diseases. The half-life of Factor IX has been reported to range from 18 to 24 hours.[7]

For indications and treatment, see Chapter 4: Hemostatic Disorders.

Other Recombinant and Plasma Protein Derivatives

Antithrombin Concentrate

Antithrombin (AT) is an important inhibitor of coagulation and inflammation. Thrombin and activated Factors IX, X, XI, and XII are inhibited by AT. The rate at which these factors are inhibited is dramatically increased in the presence of heparin. Congenital deficiencies of AT are associated with venous thrombotic disease.[11] AT concentrates are prepared from pooled units of human plasma from normal donors and are used to treat patients with hereditary AT deficiency who have thrombosis or who require prophylaxis when they are scheduled to undergo surgical or obstetric procedures. A recombinant AT product (Atryn, GTC Biotherapeutics, Framingham, MA) is now licensed in the United States for the prevention of perioperative and peripartum thromboembolic events in hereditary antithrombin-deficient patients. The recombinant protein has a different glycosylation pattern resulting in greater heparin affinity, but the novel epitopes could potentially induce an immune response in recipients. The plasma half-life of the recombinant product is considerably shorter than the plasma-derived product (10.5 vs 60 hours).[12]

Recombinant Factor VIIa and aPCCs

Recombinant Factor VIIa (NovoSeven, NovoNordisk, Bagsvaerd, Denmark) (rFVIIa) is licensed to treat and prevent bleeding episodes in patients with an inhibitor to Factor VIII or Factor IX (either acquired or with hemophilia A or B) and in patients with congenital Factor VII deficiency.[13] rFVIIa interacts with tissue factor, binds to surfaces of activated platelets, and directly activates Factor X. Activated Factor X complexes with Factor Va, a process that leads to a thrombin burst and clot formation. The resulting shortened prothrombin time (PT) does not predict clinical effectiveness. rFVIIa has a mean half-life of 2.7 hours. This product has been used off-label to treat patients with myriad bleeding problems, including platelet function disorders, liver disease, intracranial hemorrhage, trauma, postpartum hemorrhage, and reversal of anticoagulant agents. Anecdotal reports have demonstrated efficacy in many of these clinical situations, but many failures also occur, and the few well-controlled trials that have been conducted have generally been disappointing.[13,14] The most appropriate dose and schedule for treating any indication is not fully established, and this product should be used in consultation with a physician who is experienced in its use. Adverse effects include a risk of venous and arterial thromboembolic events.[15]

Activated prothrombin complex concentrates (aPCCs) contain activated Factors II, VII, and X. These factors are also able to bypass an inhibitor to Factor VIII or IX to achieve hemostasis. This product is derived from heat-treated human plasma. The choice of product (rFVIIa vs aPCCs) to treat an inhibitor depends on the type and current titer of the inhibitor, the location of the bleeding, and previous response to these products.[1]

Fibrinogen Concentrate

Fibrinogen concentrate (RiaSTAP, CSL Behring, King of Prussia, PA) is a pasteurized human product stored as a lyophilized powder at room temperature. Vials contain 900 to 1300 mg fibrinogen. Fibrinogen Concentrate is indicated for the treatment of acute bleeding episodes in patients with congenital fibrinogen deficiency, including afibrinogenemia and hypofibrinogenemia.

Protein C Concentrate

Protein C is a vitamin-K-dependent inhibitor of coagulation that is converted to its active form by the thrombin/thrombomodulin complex.[16] Human-plasma-derived protein C concentrate (Ceprotin, Baxter Healthcare, Westlake Village, CA) is available for treatment of patients with severe congenital protein C deficiency. Recombinant human-activated protein C (Xigris, Eli Lilly, Indianapolis, IN) has been shown to reduce mortality rates in septic patients with a high risk of death; however, it is associated with an increased risk of bleeding. Ongoing studies are needed to define which patients are most likely to benefit from this therapy.[17,18]

Fibrin Sealant

Fibrin sealants (also called fibrin glue) consist of concentrated fibrinogen and thrombin, which on mixing create a fibrin clot. Fibrin sealant has been used in a diverse number of surgical procedures as a hemostat, sealant, and adhesive; the most extensive use has been in cardiothoracic surgery and neurosurgery.[19,20] The Food and Drug Administration (FDA) has licensed multiple commercially prepared fibrin sealant kits that use lyophilized, virus-inactivated human fibrinogen and thrombin. Cryoprecipitate can also be used as a source of fibrinogen. A commercial kit has the benefit of standardized preparation and ease of administration, as well as a low risk of virus transmission. Bovine thrombin preparations may contain bovine Factor V, which can result in the formation of antibodies that cross-react with human Factor V and lead to serious clinical sequelae. Both recombinant and plasma-derived human thrombin products are also available.

Factor XIII Concentrate

The first Factor XIII concentrate, Corifact (CSL Behring, King of Prussia, PA), has been approved in the United States and is known as Fibrogammin P in other countries. It is indicated for routine prophylactic treatment of congenital Factor XIII deficiency. In addition, Factor XIII concentrate has also been shown to improve clot stability when used in conjunction with rFVIIa in hemophilia A patients with inhibitors.[21] The half-life of plasma-derived Factor XIII is approximately 9 days, and Corifact is dosed every 28 days. If concentrates are unavailable, patients are typically given plasma or cryoprecipitate. A recombinant Factor XIII is also in development.

Albumin and Plasma Protein Fraction

Description of Products

Albumin is derived from human plasma and composed of 96% albumin and 4% globulin and other proteins. It is prepared by the cold alcohol fractionation process and subsequently heated to 60 C for 10 hours to prevent viral disease transmission. Plasma protein fraction (PPF) is a similar product, except that it is subjected to fewer purification steps in the fractionation process. PPF contains about 83% albumin and 17% globulin. Normal serum albumin is available as a 25% or a 5% solution, while PPF is available as a 5% solution. Each of the products has a sodium content of about 145 mmol/L (145 mEq/L). The 5% albumin solution is osmotically and oncotically equivalent to plasma and the 25% solution has osmotic and oncotic effects that are five times those of plasma. Albumin has a plasma half-life of 15 to 20 days. These products contain no coagulation factors.

Indications

Albumin is used for its oncotic activity in patients who are both hypovolemic and hypoproteinemic (eg, in clinical settings of shock, thermal injury, nephrotic syndrome, and large-volume paracentesis). It is also used as a replacement fluid in patients undergoing therapeutic plasma exchange.[22] However, the specific clinical situations for which albumin therapy is recommended and in which it has proved to be beneficial remain a subject of controversy. A large study comparing albumin to saline for fluid resuscitation in the intensive care unit found no adverse effect of albumin and found similar outcomes with the use of albumin or normal saline for fluid resuscitation.[23] Another meta-analysis found that albumin can bestow benefit in diverse clinical settings such as during cardiac surgery, hypoalbuminemia, ascites, sepsis, and burn care.[24] Indications for the use of PPF parallel those given for 5% albumin.

Contraindications and Precautions

Albumin is not indicated for correction of hypoproteinemia or nutritional hypoalbuminemia. Albumin administration in patients with traumatic brain injury has been associated with higher mortality rates than saline.[25] Use of the 25% albumin solution is contraindicated in dehydrated patients unless it is supplemented by the infusion of crystalloid solutions to provide volume expansion. The 25% albumin solution can be diluted only with normal saline or D5W; sterile water should not be used. Reported side effects include flushing, urticaria, chills, fever, and headache. Rapid infusion of PPF at rates higher than 10 mL/minute has produced hypotension attributed to the presence of both sodium acetate and Hageman factor (Factor XII) fragments.[26] PPF, but not albumin, is contraindicated for intra-arterial administration or infusion during cardiopulmonary bypass. Albumin and PPF are extremely safe in regard to transmission of viruses.

Dose and Administration

Albumin and PPF need not be given through a filter. Treatment of hypotension with albumin and PPF should be guided by the patient's hemodynamic response. A 500-mL dose (10-20 mL/kg or 0.5-1 g/kg/dose in children) is given rapidly for shock. In the absence of symptomatic hypovolemia, an infusion rate of 1 to 2 mL/minute is suitable. In burn patients, the dose of albumin or PPF is the amount necessary to maintain the circulating plasma protein level at 5.2 g/dL or higher. Albumin will not correct chronic hypoalbuminemia and should not be used for long-term therapy.

Synthetic Volume Expanders

Description of Products

Crystalloid solutions such as normal saline and lactated Ringer's solution are isotonic with plasma. Normal saline contains only sodium and chloride ions, while lactated Ringer's solution also contains potassium, calcium, and lactate. Hypotonic solutions of sodium chloride are also available. Crystalloid solutions are less expensive than the colloid solutions.

The most common colloid used for volume expansion is hydroxyethyl starch (HES). HES is available as a 6% solution in normal saline. The intravascular half-life of HES is more than 24 hours. Other plasma expanders, such as gelatins and dextran are also available.

Indications

By virtue of their oncotic properties, colloids are useful as volume expanders in the treatment of hemorrhagic shock and burns. Crystalloid solutions alone expand the plasma volume temporarily as they rapidly cross capillary membranes, but only one-third of the salt solution remains in the intravascular space.[27] Accordingly, two to three volumes of crystalloid are required to replace one volume of lost plasma. Crystalloid and colloid solutions are relatively nontoxic and inexpensive, are readily available, can be stored at room temperature, require no compatibility testing, and are free of the risk of transfusion-transmitted disease. The relative merits of crystalloid and colloid solutions for acute hypovolemia remain a subject of controversy.[28,29] A meta-analysis conducted to compare the effects of different colloid solutions found no evidence that one solution is more effective than any other.[30]

Contraindications and Precautions

Circulatory overload is a risk associated with all volume expanders. The side effects associated with HES occur less frequently than do those associated with dextran, but the side effects of HES do include prolongation of PT and activated partial thromboplastin time (aPTT) as well as pruritus. Dextran can produce anaphylactic reactions, fever, rash, tachycardia, hypotension, as well as increased bleeding tendencies resulting from its interference with platelet function and its stimulation of fibrinolysis. Renal failure has also been reported with the infusion of low-molecular-weight dextran products. High-molecular-weight dextrans have been known to aggregate red cells in vitro, leading to interference with blood typing and crossmatching.

Administration

Crystalloid and colloid solutions do not have to be administered through a blood filter.

Immune Globulin

Description of Products

Immune globulins are prepared by cold ethanol fractionation from pools of human plasma from 15,000 to 60,000 healthy volunteers. Gamma globulin preparations and specific hyperimmune globulin preparations with high titers against specific infectious agents or toxins are available for intramuscular (IM) use. These products have a number of disadvantages: IM administration requires 4 to 7 days to achieve peak plasma levels; the maximum dose that can be given is limited by muscle mass; administration may be painful; and IM immune globulin (IMIG) can undergo proteolytic breakdown at the IM site. IM products are now given primarily for disease prophylaxis. These preparations are sterile solutions with protein concentrations of approximately 16.5 g/dL. The predominant immune globulin is IgG, but IgA and IgM may also be present.

Intravenous (IV) immune globulin (IVIG) minimizes some of the disadvantages of IMIG. Sterile, lyophilized IVIG differs from IMIG in the mode of preparation, use of additives, pH, and protein content (stated on the package insert). More than 90% of the protein is IgG; there are only trace quantities of IgA and IgM. Infusion of IVIG products can achieve peak levels of IgG immediately after infusion. The gamma globulin molecules of IVIG preparations are intact. IVIG contains antibodies to a wide variety of infectious agents, but specific titers are not known for most preparations. The half-lives of IVIG and IMIG preparations vary from 18 to 32 days, which is the same range as that for native IgG.[31,32]

Indications

Immune globulin preparations can be used to provide passive antibody prophylaxis for susceptible persons who are exposed to certain diseases and as replacement therapy in primary immunodeficiency states. Immune globulin is also used to modulate the immune system in autoimmune diseases. Both FDA-approved and off-label, non-FDA-approved indications continue to expand. The efficacy of IVIG in various clinical settings has been extensively reviewed.[31,33-36]

Contraindications and Precautions

Adverse reactions to immune globulin preparations include headache, fatigue, chills, backache, lightheadedness, fever, flushing, and nausea. An IgA-depleted product is available and has been used safely in IgA-deficient patients with anti-IgA.[37] IM preparations must not be given intravenously because they contain immunoglobulin aggregates that may activate the complement and kinin systems. Infectious risk is effectively mitigated using virus inactivation techniques. Passive transfer of blood group antibodies may produce a positive direct antiglobulin test (DAT) result in recipients. Clinically significant hemolysis may occur on rare occasions. Renal dysfunction and acute renal failure have been reported with sucrose-containing IVIG preparations, and these products should be given with caution to patients at risk for developing acute renal failure.[38] Information about management of infusion rate is included in the package insert; these recommendations should be stringently followed because some data suggest that too rapid an infusion of this hyperviscous product may increase the risk of renal damage and thrombosis.

Dose and Administration

The dose depends on the reason for administration, patient characteristics, and the preparation used (IM or IV).

Rh Immune Globulin

Description of Product

Rh Immune Globulin (RhIG) is prepared from pooled human plasma and marketed under the trade names of WinRho SDF (Cangene, Winnipeg, Canada), Rhophylac (CSL Behring, King of Prussia, PA), and RhoGAM (Ortho-Clinical Diagnostics, Raritan, NJ). RhIG contains mostly IgG anti-D. Various dosages are available for either IM or IV administration (WinRho and Rhophylac). RhoGAM is available in 300-µg (1500 IU) and 50-µg (150 IU) (microdose) preparations for IM injection only and is used for the prevention of alloimmunization to the D antigen. Solvent/detergent-treated IV preparations are approved by the FDA for both suppression of immunization to the D antigen and treatment of immune thrombocytopenia. The package insert should be consulted for dosing recommendations for all products. These preparations appear to be very safe with respect to infectious disease transmission. The availability of a safe and effective monoclonal anti-D IgG, which could be produced in limitless quantities, would be very desirable. However, experiments with monoclonal anti-D for Rh prophylaxis have not been successful so far.

Indications and Dosage

Antepartum Prevention of Alloimmunization to the D Antigen

For D-negative females, a 50-µg microdose of RhIG can be used in the situations of abortion, miscarriage, and termination of ectopic pregnancy occurring during the first 12 weeks of gestation (fetal red cell mass at 12 weeks of gestation is estimated to be <2.5 mL). After 12 weeks of gestation, a full dose (300-µg) of IM or IV RhIG should be administered for these indications. A full dose is also recommended for use after amniocentesis and for any other obstetric complication (eg, abdominal trauma and antepartum hemorrhage) or obstetric manipulation (eg, external version) occurring after 12 weeks of pregnancy.[39,40] RhIG should be given (preferably) within 72 hours of amniocentesis or any other obstetric event that may cause fetomaternal hemorrhage (FMH), including termination of pregnancy, unless it has been determined either that the fetus is D negative or that maternal immunization to the D antigen has already occurred. If repeated amniocenteses are performed, additional doses should be considered, particularly if the procedures are performed more than 21 days apart.

All nonimmunized D-negative females should receive antepartum prophylaxis with a full dose of either IM or IV RhIG at 28 weeks of gestation. Together, postpartum prophylaxis and antepartum prophylaxis have reduced the number of D-negative females who become alloimmunized to the D antigen during gestation to 0.1%; the rate with postpartum prophylaxis alone was 1% to 2%.[41]

Postpartum Prevention of Alloimmunization to the D Antigen

All D-negative females who deliver D-positive infants should receive at least a 300-µg dose of IM or IV RhIG unless previous maternal immunization to the D antigen, not related to antepartum RhIG therapy, has been demonstrated. If the result of the infant's typing is questionable, RhIG should be given to the mother. A postpartum maternal blood sample must be drawn and evaluated for the extent of FMH. If the screening test for FMH is positive, hemorrhage must be quantified to assess the need for additional doses of RhIG. This is usually accomplished by performing a Kleihauer-Betke test or a flow cytometric assay. A full dose (300 µg) of RhIG protects against alloimmunization to the D antigen after exposure of up to 15 mL of D-positive red cells. In about 1 in 300 deliveries, the FMH exceeds 15 mL of red cells, and one or more additional doses of RhIG are required. In this setting, IV RhIG may prove to be a convenient alternative to multiple IM injections. RhIG should be administered to the mother within 72 hours of delivery. However, if more than 72 hours have elapsed, the dose should still be given, as it may yet protect against maternal alloimmunization. Antepartum administration may cause a positive antibody screen in the mother because of passively acquired antibody. Antepartum RhIG has been associated with weakly reactive DAT results in the newborn, but this is not associated with clinical evidence of hemolysis. Obtaining a careful patient history is essential in determining the likely cause of anti-D in the pregnant or postpartum female. Because administration of anti-D to D-negative individuals carries minimal risk, RhIG should always be given when there is any question about whether the anti-D is caused by passive or active immunization.

Special Considerations

The package insert should be followed carefully for determination of dose for any indication. RhIG may also be used when D-positive blood components are given to D-negative females of childbearing potential and to children. A 300-µg dose is sufficient to protect against the immunizing effect of the D-positive red cells contained in platelet products, although this practice may not be necessary for a single dose of D-positive apheresis platelets.[42] The administration of multiple vials of IM RhIG after the transfusion of D-positive red cells is generally impractical. IV RhIG is more suitable than IM RhIG for this purpose, but the use of either must be weighed against the risk of inducing clinically significant hemolysis in the recipient. IV RhIG may also be an important alternative to IM therapy in patients with coagulopathy and significant thrombocytopenia. An 18-μg dose of IV RhIG should be given within 72 hours for each milliliter of red cells transfused. Some have advocated the use of red cell exchange transfusion in addition to IV RhIG when large amounts of D-positive red cells have been transfused to a D-negative recipient.

IV RhIG is approved by the FDA for use in D-positive patients with ITP who have not undergone splenectomy.[43] The initial dose is 50 to 75 μg/kg unless the hemoglobin is less than 10 g/dL, in which case 25 to 40 μg/kg is recommended. Depending on the initial response, additional doses may be required. The primary advantages of IV RhIG over IVIG in the treatment of ITP are the lower cost and lower volume of IV RhIG. There is a risk of red cell hemolysis, and the patient's hemoglobin level should be monitored.

References

1. Medical and Scientific Advisory Council. MASAC recommendations concerning products licensed for the treatment of hemophilia and other bleeding disorders. MASAC Document 195. New York: National Hemophilia Foundation, 2010.
2. Pipe S. Consideration in hemophilia therapy selection. Semin Hematol 2006;43(2 Suppl):S23-7.
3. Franchini M. Plasma-derived versus recombinant factor VIII concentrates for the treatment of haemophilia A: Recombinant is better. Blood Transfus 2010;8:292-6.
4. Mannucci PM. Plasma-derived versus recombinant factor VIII concentrates for the treatment of haemophilia A: plasma-derived is better. Blood Transfus 2010;8:288-91.

5. Brettler DB, Forsberg AD, Levine PH, et al. Factor VIII:C concentrate purified from plasma using monoclonal antibodies: Human studies. Blood 1989;73:1859-63.

6. Luban NL. The spectrum of safety: A review of the safety of current hemophilia products. Semin Hematol 2003;40(3 Suppl):10-15.

7. Montgomery RR, Gill JC, Scott JP. Hemophilia and von Willebrand disease. In: Nathan DG, Orkin SH, Ginsburg D, et al, eds. Nathan and Oski's hematology of infancy and childhood. 7th ed, vol. 2. Philadelphia: WB Saunders, 2009: 1547-76.

8. Takabe K, Holman PR, Herbst KD, et al. Successful perioperative management of factor X deficiency associated with primary amyloidosis. J Gastrointest Surg 2004;8:358-62.

9. Franchini M, Lippi G. Prothrombin complex concentrates: an update. Blood Transfus 2010;8:149-54.

10. Leissinger CA, Blatt PM, Hoots WK, et al. Role of prothrombin complex concentrates in reversing warfarin anticoagulation: A review of the literature. Am J Hematol 2008; 83:137-43.

11. Menache D, Grossman BJ, Jackson CM. Antithrombin III: Physiology, deficiency and replacement therapy. Transfusion 1992;32:580-8.

12. Maclean P, Tait RC. Hereditary and acquired antithrombin deficiency. Drugs 2007;67:1429-40.

13. Grottke O, Henzler D, Rossaint R. Activated recombinant factor VII (rFVIIa). Best Pract Res Clin Anaesthesiology 2010;24:95-106.

14. Stanworth SJ, Birchall J, Doree CJ, et al. Recombinant factor VIIa for the prevention and treatment of bleeding in patients without haemophilia. Cochrane Database Syst Rev 2007;(2):CD005011.

15. Levi M, Levy JH, Andersen HF, Truloff D. Safety of recombinant activated Factor VII in randomized clinical trials. N Engl J Med 2010;363:1791-800.

16. Griffin JH, Fernandez JA, Gale AJ, et al. Activated protein C. J Thromb Haemost 2007;5(Suppl 1):73-80.

17. Bernard GR, Vincent JL, Laterre PF, et al for the PROW-ESS study group. Efficacy and safety of recombinant human activated protein C for severe sepsis. N Engl J Med 2001;344:699-709.

18. DeBacker D. Benefit-risk assessment of drotrecogin alfa (activated) in the treatment of sepsis. Drug Saf 2007;30: 995-1010.

19. Spotnitz WD, Burks S. Hemostats, sealants, and adhesives II: Update as well as how and when to use the components of the surgical toolbox. Clin Appl Thromb Hemost 2010; 16:497-514.

20. Albala DM, Lawson JH. Recent clinical and investigational applications of fibrin sealant in selected surgical special-ties. J Am Coll Surg 2006;202:685-97.

21. Rea CJ, Foley JH, Ingerslev J, Sorensen B. Factor XIII combined with recombinant factor VIIa: A new means of treating severe haemophilia A. J Thromb Haemost 2011;9: 510-16.

22. Erstad BL, Gales BJ, Rappaport WD. The use of albumin in clinical practice. Arch Intern Med 1991;151:901-11.

23. The SAFE Study Investigators. A comparison of albumin and saline for fluid resuscitation in the intensive care unit. N Engl J Med 2004;350:2247-56.

24. Haynes GR, Navickis RJ, Wiles MM. Albumin administra-tion—what is the evidence of clinical benefit? A system-atic review of randomized controlled trials. Eur J Anaesthesiol 2003;20:771-93.

25. The SAFE Study Investigators. Saline or albumin for fluid resuscitation in patients with traumatic brain injury. N Engl J Med 2007;357:874-84.

26. Olinger GN, Werner PH, Boncheck LI, et al. Vasodilator effects of the sodium acetate in pooled protein fraction. Ann Surg 1979;190:305-11.

27. Cervera AL, Moss G. Crystalloid distribution following hemorrhage and hemodilution: Mathematical model and

prediction of optimum volumes for equilibration at normo-volemia. J Trauma 1974;14:506-20.

28. Bagshaw SM, Bellomo R. The influence of volume management on outcome. Curr Opin Crit Care 2007;13:541-8.

29. Perel P, Roberts I. Colloids versus crystalloids for fluid resuscitation in critically ill patients. Cochrane Database Syst Rev 1997;(4):CD000567.

30. Bunn F, Trivedi D, Ashraf S. Colloid solutions for fluid resuscitation. Cochrane Database Syst Rev 2008;(1): CD001319.

31. Knezevic-Maramica I, Kruskall MS. Intravenous immune globulins: An update for clinicians. Transfusion 2003;43: 1460-80.

32. Ršmer J, Morgenthaler JJ, Scherz R, et al. Characterization of various immunoglobulin preparations for intravenous application 1. Protein composition and antibody content. Vox Sang 1982;42:62-73.

33. Kotlan B, Stroncek DF, Marincola FM. Intravenous immunoglobulin-based immunotherapy: An arsenal of possibilities for patients and science. Immunotherapy 2009;1:995-1015.

34. Anderson D, Ali K, Blanchette V, et al. Guidelines on the use of intravenous immune globulin for hematologic conditions. Transfus Med Rev 2007;21(Suppl 1):S9-S56.

35. NIH consensus development conference. Intravenous immunoglobulin: Prevention and treatment of disease. JAMA 1990;264:3189-93.

36. Cowden J, Parker SK. Intravenous immunoglobulin production, uses and side effects. Pediatr Infect Dis J 2006; 25:641-2.

37. Cunningham-Rundles C, Zhou Z, Mankarious S, et al. Long-term use of IgA-depleted intravenous immunoglobulin in immunodeficient subjects with anti-IgA antibodies. J Clin Immunol 1993;13:272-8.

38. Pierce LR, Jain N. Risks associated with the use of intravenous immunoglobulin. Transfus Med Rev 2003;17:241-51.

39. American College of Obstetrics and Gynecology. Prevention of Rho(D) isoimmunization. ACOG Practice Bull 1999;4:1-8.
40. Hartwell EA. Use of Rh immune globulin: ASCP practice parameter. Am J Clin Pathol 1998;110:281-92.
41. Bowman J. Thirty-five years of Rh prophylaxis. Transfusion 2003;43:1661-6.
42. Bartley AN, Carpenter JB, Berg MP. D+ platelet transfusions in D– patients: Cause for concern? Immunohematology 2009;25:5-8.
43. Sandler SG, Tutuncuoglu SO. Immune thrombocytopenic purpura—current management practices. Expert Opin Pharmacother 2004;5:2515-27.

TRANSFUSION PRACTICES

Surgical Blood Ordering Practices

Most healthy adult patients with a normal hemoglobin level who undergo elective surgical procedures do not require blood replacement if there is blood loss of less than 1000 mL, provided that intravascular volume is maintained with crystalloid or colloid solutions. In fact, only a small percentage of all surgical patients actually receive blood transfusions. Several methods are available to most appropriately order blood for surgery.

Maximum Surgical Blood Order Schedule

When a blood transfusion is anticipated for routine surgery, only about 16% of the patients actually receive a blood transfusion.[1] However, blood reserved for surgical patients is removed from the general inventory and is unavailable to other patients. If unused after a day or more, the blood is returned to the general inventory, and the expiration date will have been effectively shortened by the time in reserve. Preoperative blood ordering schedules are used to predict surgical blood needs and efficiently allocate blood on the day of surgery. A review of institutional blood use over time can be used to derive a maximum surgical blood order schedule (MSBOS) that would account for 90% of the blood needs for a particular surgery.[2] A MSBOS also serves to reduce pretransfusion testing, avoid outdating of blood units, and provide a guide for autologous blood collection. A MSBOS can be developed by analyzing blood usage for common elective surgical procedures and comparing the number of Red Blood Cell (RBC) units that are crossmatched to the number of units that are transfused. The development and acceptance of blood order schedules for elective surgery require a close working relationship among the transfusion, surgery, and anesthesiology services. In some institutions, the MSBOS may require the approval of the hospital transfusion committee or its equivalent.

Blood ordering practices can be monitored through the crossmatch-to-transfusion (C:T) ratio for a particular procedure or surgeon, and the information can be used to develop preoperative blood order schedules. Tracking of the C:T ratio helps to decrease overestimates of the need for crossmatched blood and can identify procedures that may benefit from more targeted blood schedules. Nationally, a C:T ratio of less than 2 is considered appropriate for blood units ordered and crossmatched.

Type and Screen

A type and screen (T/S) order involves typing the patient's red cells for ABO and Rh type and screening the patient's serum for clinically significant red cell alloantibodies. These are antibodies capable of causing red cell destruction after transfusion of incompatible red cells. A T/S order is recommended for surgical procedures with minimal blood loss, which is defined as procedures requiring no blood transfusion in 90% of cases. When the antibody screen is negative, no clinically significant red cell antibodies are identified and no blood is reserved for the patient. When the screen is positive, clinically significant antibodies may be present and the T/S is converted to a type and crossmatch (T/C). The blood bank will proceed with antibody identification and obtain 1 to 2 units of antigen-negative RBCs. These units will be crossmatched and reserved for the patient.[3(p35)]

Type and Crossmatch

A T/C is the same as a T/S except that blood is selected and reserved for the patient. A T/C is ordered when red cell transfusion is anticipated. For surgical procedures, a T/C is ordered for procedures that require transfusion in 90% of cases.

If the antibody screen is negative and no clinically significant red cell antibodies are identified, an electronic crossmatch or a rapid serologic crossmatch can be performed (see Fig 1). The manual rapid crossmatch serves only to confirm ABO compatibility between the patient and the unit. In many hospitals, the rapid crossmatch has been replaced with an electronic crossmatch, in which ABO and Rh compatibility are confirmed and units are crossmatched using computer software.[3(p36),4] For patients with a negative antibody screen, ABO-specific crossmatched blood can be available in 10 to 15 minutes.

If the patient's serum contains clinically significant red cell antibodies, an antiglobulin crossmatch is mandatory[3(p35)] and will require an additional 30 to 40 minutes to complete before units can be released for transfusion. By proactively converting a T/S to a T/C when unexpected antibodies are detected in the preoperative antibody screen, the blood bank ensures that crossmatched blood (usually 1-2 units) will be available during surgery within the 10- to 15-minute time frame. The proactive conversion to a T/C safeguards the patient against unexpected delays in blood delivery.

Delays may occur when patients who are to undergo surgery are admitted to the hospital on the day of surgery, because the blood bank may not have sufficient time to identify a clinically significant antibody and then find crossmatch-compatible units. This process takes a minimum of 90 minutes to complete for patients with a simple antibody, and can take hours to days in complicated cases. To prevent this delay, patients should have blood specimens drawn for compatibility testing well in advance of the need for blood, particularly for patients with a history of blood exposure from pregnancy, surgery, or transfusion. The 72-hour limit for drawing a preoperative T/S sample can be

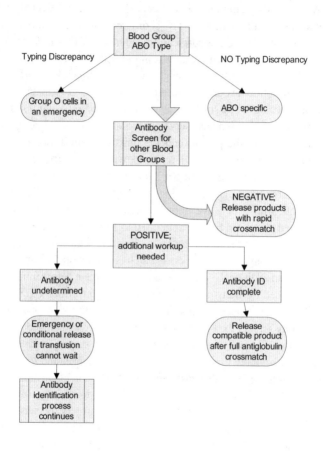

Figure 1. Sample processing for ABO type, antibody screen, and crossmatch *[Courtesy Roberta Arney, MT(ASCP)SBB].*

extended for patients with a negative antibody screen and a history of no transfusion or pregnancy within the preceding 3 months. In these patients, samples can be drawn up to 1 month from the time of surgery.[5] This is not true for patients with a positive screen or a history of a clinically significant alloantibody. In these patients, a current blood specimen is required to cross-match units for surgery.[3(p35)]

Alternatives to Allogeneic Blood Transfusion

Every reasonable effort should be made to transfuse blood judiciously. Some patients who refuse donated blood because of religious or other beliefs may accept alternatives to allogeneic blood transfusion. All patients undergoing elective surgical procedures for which blood replacement is anticipated should be considered as candidates for a preoperative blood management program as part of an integrated effort to limit exposure to allogeneic blood. Strategies employed to limit allogeneic blood transfusion may include treatment of preoperative anemia, discontinuing antithrombotic and antiplatelet agents, the use of pharmacologic agents to support hematopoiesis and hemostasis, volume expanders, and autologous blood collection (pre-, intra-, and/or postoperatively).[6,7] The potential advantages of autologous blood include reduced risks of 1) infectious disease transmission; 2) febrile reactions, allergic reactions, or transfusion-associated graft-vs-host disease (TA-GVHD); and 3) alloimmunization to red cell, platelet, and leukocyte antigens. Autologous blood can also provide compatible blood for patients with alloantibodies, as well as reduce the need for allogeneic blood.[6] All participants should be familiar with every aspect of a perioperative autologous blood collection program, such as which blood components are to be collected and stored. Patients must also understand that involvement in such a program does not guarantee that they will receive a transfusion consisting exclusively of their own blood. The reason for this is that unexpected blood loss or an inability to collect the desired number of units may occur. A perioperative blood program must have defined policies and must conform to perioperative blood collection and administration standards.[8,9]

Preoperative Autologous Blood Donation

Preoperative autologous blood donation (PAD) is the process of collecting and storing the patient's own blood before surgery. The advantages of autologous blood are listed above; however, there are also disadvantages to PAD.[6,10] Autologous units are more expensive than allogeneic units and may not be reimbursed by insurance. In addition, up to 10% to 20% of patients referred for PAD are unable to successfully donate because of an underlying medical condition (2-3%) or adverse reactions and complications associated with donation (6-17%).[10,11] In one study, the rate of serious adverse reactions was 12 times higher in autologous donors than community blood donors.[12] Finally, PAD can lead to iatrogenic preoperative anemia, increasing the probability that a patient will require transfusion at the time of surgery.[6] Under a routine PAD schedule [1 unit per week without erythropoietin (EPO) supplementation], endogenous EPO increases only modestly (11-19%) and is not sufficient to support the patient's hematocrit over the course of several donations. The wastage rate for autologous blood is approximately 60%, indicating that most autologous donations are unnecessary.

Because there are no specific requirements as to age, both elderly patients and children younger than 17 years of age can participate, although the risk of adverse reactions is higher in these age groups.[6,11] For patients weighing less than 110 pounds, it is advisable to limit the volume of blood drawn at each donation to 10% of the patient's total blood volume.[6,13] Autologous collection during pregnancy can be performed safely, but it is usually unnecessary. PAD is not recommended for patients undergoing procedures with a low probability (<10%) of requiring transfusion.[6]

Certain guidelines for autologous donors are less stringent than those for volunteer donors. The hematocrit should be at least 33% (hemoglobin 11.0 g/dL) before donation.[3(35)] Potential autologous donors who are anemic should be evaluated by a physician to determine the cause of anemia before the first unit is drawn. Concurrent medical problems can exclude some candidates from PAD, and criteria for exclusion may vary among facilities. Contraindications to PAD include infection or risk of bacteremia, active seizure disorder, uncontrolled hypertension, aortic stenosis, recent myocardial infarction and stroke, and severe cardiopulmonary disease.[6,7,10]

The transfusion of autologous blood is not without risk. The risks of a patient's receipt of the wrong unit, bacterial contamination, and volume overload are similar to the risks for allogeneic blood.[6,10] Because mortality from allogeneic blood transfusion is more likely caused by administrative error than by transfusion-transmitted infection, the more severe risks of autologous transfusion now approach those of allogeneic transfusion.[6] In addition, patients who donate blood preoperatively are more likely to receive a transfusion, which increases the potential for administration errors.[10] The decision to transfuse a patient should not be based on the availability of autologous blood, but rather should be based on the same considerations as allogeneic blood transfusion. This more conservative approach will mitigate the more severe risks of transfusion.

Acute Normovolemic Hemodilution

Another form of autologous transfusion is acute normovolemic hemodilution (ANH), which refers to the collection of 1 or more Whole Blood units at the onset of surgery and reinfusion at the end of the procedure. To prevent hypotension, the volume of blood that is removed is replaced with crystalloid or colloid solutions.[6] This technique is most useful in patients with an adequate preoperative hemoglobin level (>10.0 g/dL) and no severe myocardial disease, who are undergoing procedures associated with large-volume blood loss (1000-1500 mL). Relative contraindications for ANH are severe anemia, active ischemic cardiac disease, a low cardiac ejection fraction (<30%), known coagulopathy, and underlying hemoglobinopathy.[6,7] ANH is considered acceptable by many, but not all, Jehovah's Witness patients.

ANH has several advantages over PAD. Following ANH, blood lost during surgery has a lower hematocrit and viscosity, which conserves red cell mass and may improve perfusion to capillary beds. In addition, the reinfused blood provides a source of fresh platelets and clotting factors, which may have been depleted during surgery. Finally, ANH is more cost effective than PAD, by eliminating the costs associated with testing, inventory management, and wastage.[6]

The techniques used for ANH must ensure that the blood is collected in a sterile manner and is properly labeled and stored in approved plastic blood-collection bags. Units of blood can be stored at room temperature for as long as 8 hours from the start of collection or at 1 to 6 C for as long as 24 hours from the start of collection, provided 1 to 6 C storage was begun within 8 hours of initiating the collection.[8] Close patient monitoring is required to guard against fluid overload.

Intraoperative Blood Recovery

Intraoperative blood recovery involves the collection and subsequent reinfusion of blood recovered from the operative site or from an extracorporeal circuit.[9] It is often used in conjunction with other blood management interventions.[6,14] Patients can receive their own shed blood, which can decrease the need for allogeneic blood transfusion by 23% to 54%.[14] This technique should be considered when estimated blood loss is 20% or more of the patient's blood volume and the mean transfusion for the procedure exceeds 1 unit. Relative contraindications are infection, malignancy, hemoglobinopathies, cold agglutinins, and the presence of certain contaminants (urine, fat, amniotic fluid) or pharmacologic agents in the surgical field (hypotonic irrigation fluids, clotting agents, catecholamines).[6,9] Blood recovery has

74

been performed safely during obstetric and oncologic surgery provided blood is washed and reinfused with a leukocyte reduction filter.[9] Blood recovered by intraoperative collection cannot be transfused to other patients.

Various types of devices are available for retrieval of blood from the operative site.[14] The recovered blood should be washed and filtered before reinfusion.[9,15] The washing of shed blood is recommended to eliminate complement and other activated factors. Cell-washing devices can prepare the equivalent of 10 units of allogeneic blood per hour for reinfusion to a massively bleeding patient. Blood collected and processed under sterile conditions and washed with 0.9% saline USP can be stored as long as 4 hours from the end of collection at room temperature or as long as 24 hours from the start of collection at 1 to 6 C, provided that refrigeration was begun within 4 hours of the start of collection.[8] A written protocol describing all procedures involved must be maintained.[8,9]

Postoperative Blood Recovery

Techniques are also available for recovering blood shed postoperatively from surgical drains, chest tubes, or joint cavities. This blood is typically defibrinated and unclottable, and it contains high concentrations of fibrinogen-fibrin degradation products, cytokines, activated complement, and cellular proteases.[6,14,15] In addition, postoperative blood shed from drains is extremely hemodiluted and contains partially hemolyzed red cells. The utility of this technique remains controversial and is limited by both the volume and hematocrit of the shed blood.

The collected blood can be processed with or without cell washing, but the washing of shed blood is preferred to eliminate complement and other activated factors.[15] Shed blood must be filtered before reinfusion. Blood intended for reinfusion must be given within 6 hours of the start of collection.[8] Postoperative blood recovery is contraindicated in the presence of local or systemic infection.

Directed Blood Donations

Directed blood donations can supply red cells, platelets, plasma, or cryoprecipitate to a specific patient. Directed donors must meet the same eligibility guidelines as volunteer blood donors. Medical indications for directed donations include red cells with an unusual phenotype, HLA-compatible platelets or granulocytes, and the desire to limit donor exposures in a patient with a predictable transfusion requirement. State laws may also mandate that patients be offered the opportunity to procure directed blood donors.

Relatives and friends of patients may be highly motivated to donate blood for compassionate reasons or because of a perception of increased safety. There is no evidence to suggest that directed blood donations are safer than volunteer donations. In addition, there is concern that some donors may feel social pressure to donate and be reluctant to acknowledge potential risk factors or underlying medical problems that would exclude them from donating blood. Recent data showed higher infectious disease positivity rates among first-time donors, which would also apply to those directed donors who are giving for the first time.[16] Directed donations from blood relatives must be irradiated to prevent TA-GVHD.[3(p38)] With rare medical exceptions, mothers should be avoided as directed donors for their children because of the increased potential risk of transfusion-related acute lung injury (TRALI) by maternal HLA antibodies.

Urgent and Massive Transfusion

Urgent Transfusion

Urgent transfusion refers to the administration of blood components (typically RBC units) before the completion of standard pretransfusion testing, when a delay in transfusion may imperil the patient. Implicit is the understanding that it is necessary to reestablish both oxygen-carrying capacity and intravascular volume. In hypovolemic shock, most authorities recommend immediate restoration of volume with crystalloid or colloid solutions. If volume replacement leads to clinical stabilization, transfusion is less urgent and should await the completion of compatibility testing. If transfusion is necessary before completion of compatibility testing, group O RBCs should be used. Whenever possible, D-negative RBCs should be used for females of childbearing potential and children to avoid the possibility of sensitization to the D antigen. Either before or after the uncrossmatched blood is issued, the patient's physician must sign a statement indicating the nature of the emergency. If the patient's screen for unexpected red cell antibodies is negative, the transfusion of uncrossmatched but now group-specific RBCs carries a very low risk of incompatibility.[17] However, this safety margin depends on the correct identification of the patient, the pretransfusion blood sample, and the blood components to be infused. Guidelines for conditions under which it is safe to switch the patient to type-specific blood are available.[3(pp40-41)]

Massive Transfusion

Massive transfusion is defined as the replacement of one or more blood volumes within 24 hours. A blood volume is estimated as 70 mL/kg or about 5000 mL (10 or more Whole Blood units) in a 70-kg adult. Patients requiring massive transfusion frequently develop multiple complications related to hypovolemia, hypothermia, tissue ischemia, dilutional coagulopathy, and acid-base disturbances.[18-20] Many patients who require massive transfusion develop a coagulopathy, but not all develop diffuse microvascular bleeding as a result.[19,20] Shock and systemic hypoperfusion contribute significantly to the development of coagulopathy and are poor prognostic indicators.[19] In trauma patients, hypoperfusion leads to systemic anticoagulation due to upregulation of thrombomodulin, generation of activated protein C, and increased fibrinolytic activity.[19,20] Hypothermia (core temperature <34C) and acidemia (pH<7.2) can also impair clotting.[20] Finally, large volumes of cold, citrated blood components can also lead to hypothermia, metabolic defects, and organ dysfunction.[10,18]

The coagulopathy of massive transfusion may be characterized by thrombocytopenia, hypofibrinogenemia, and the prolongation of prothrombin time (PT) and the activated partial thromboplastin time (aPTT). In trauma, a prolonged aPTT and base deficit >6 mEq/L are cited as useful markers of hyoperfusion, low protein C levels, and acute coagulopathy.[19,20] One disadvantage of PT and aPTT is the time required for routine testing (20-60 minutes) and their limited focus on the intrinsic and extrinsic clotting cascades (see Chapter 4: Hemostatic Disorders). As a result, whole blood clotting measurements, such as thromboelastography (TEG) and rotational TEG (RoTEG), are used by some centers in trauma and other massive transfusion settings (cardiac surgery, liver transplant) to guide transfusion therapy. [21]

Massive transfusion may be an indication for the use of Whole Blood, but Whole Blood is not usually available outside of military settings. RBCs administered with crystalloid or colloid solutions are equally effective in restoring blood volume and oxygen-carrying capacity,[22] although large volumes (>3 liters) can contribute to a dilutional coagulopathy.[18,21] To avoid exacerbating hypothermia, all crystalloids and blood components should be administered via a blood warming device.

Ideally, transfusion of plasma, platelets, and cryoprecipitate should be guided on the results of serial screening tests of hemostasis (PT, aPTT, fibrinogen, and platelet count). However, in trauma and other massive transfusion settings, it may be necessary to empirically transfuse before laboratory results are available. Many medical centers have established massive trauma protocols, in which plasma is transfused based on a predetermined RBC: plasma ratios (1:1 to 3:1). Cryoprecipitate should be administered to maintain a fibrinogen level >100 mg/dL. Platelets should be administered to maintain a platelet count of at least

50,000 to 60,000/μL. Hemostatic agents, such as desmopressin, recombinant Factor VIIa, and antifibrinolytics, can also be considered (see Chapter 4: Hemostatic Disorders).[23,24] Patients who continue to bleed despite adequate levels of platelets or coagulation factors should be thoroughly reevaluated and considered for surgical exploration.

Solid Organ Transplantation

The transplantation of solid organs, such as kidney, heart, lung, small bowel, and liver, can also present challenges for transfusion therapy. The transplant procedure and perioperative period may be associated with substantial bleeding and massive transfusion. Solid organ transplant surgeries, except kidney, typically require both RBC and plasma transfusion.

Liver and heart transplantation can be associated with massive hemorrhage.[25,26] Median blood component requirements in adult liver transplantation typically are 10 to 12 units each of RBCs, plasma, and platelets and up to 5 units of Cryoprecipitated Antihemophilic Factor (AHF).[25] Liver transplant patients often have complex preoperative coagulopathies that may be compounded during the anhepatic phase of surgery to yield profound hemostatic derangements. Normal hemostasis gradually resumes once the transplanted liver begins to function.

In general, transplanted organs are ABO compatible with the recipient. Transplantation of organs across major ABO barriers (eg, group A donor to group O recipient) can result in acute rejection and a 20% to 30% decrease in 1-year survival.[27] Protocols for transplanting across ABO in solid organ transplantation have been published.[27,28] Transplantation of major ABO-incompatible organs often requires pre- or intraoperative plasma exchange to decrease ABO antibody titers, combined with aggressive immunosuppression after the transplant procedure. Plasma products (plasma and platelets) should be selected that are compatible with both the patient's red cells and the transplanted organ. Minor ABO incompatibility is not as great a concern as major ABO incompatibility for intraoperative support; however, it can be associated with significant hemolytic anemia 10 to 21 days after surgery because of ABO (or other red cell) antibody production by passenger graft lymphocytes in the transplanted organ.[10,27]

GVHD is not commonly seen after solid organ transplantation and is usually associated with passenger lymphocytes in donor organs.[25] Because cases of TA-GVHD have occurred only rarely in this setting, the use of irradiated blood components for solid organ recipients is not routinely required (see later section on TA-GVHD).

Obstetric Transfusion Practices

Peripartum Hemorrhage

The incidence of postpartum hemorrhage (PPH) worldwide is estimated between 4% and 6% and is a leading cause of pregnancy-associated death.[29] There is no universal definition of PPH, with criteria ranging from an estimated blood loss of >500 mL per vaginal delivery, >1000 mL with cesarean delivery, a decrease in hematocrit >10%, hemodynamic instability, or need for blood transfusion. PPH can occur at delivery or may be delayed, sometimes occurring days after delivery. PPH risk factors include uterine atony, retained placenta, placenta previa and accretia, fetal death, trauma, and acquired or congenital coagulation disorders.[29]

Transfusion management of severe PPH follows the same guidelines as other instances of massive transfusion. In addition, these patients may receive pharmacologic agents to improve uterine tone. PPH that is refractory to medical and transfusion management may require uterine tamponade, uterine compression, or pelvic vessel embolization.[30]

Hemolytic Disease of Fetus and Newborn

Fetal red cells can express red cell antigens inherited from the father that may be absent in the mother. Because fetomaternal hemorrhages occur in nearly all pregnancies, a small percentage of mothers (0.06-0.24%) make antibodies against these paternally derived red cell antigens.[31] These maternal red cell alloantibodies can lead to hemolytic disease of the fetus and newborn (HDFN), in which maternal immunoglobulin G (IgG) antibodies are transported across the placenta and opsonize fetal red cells, which leads to extravascular hemolysis of fetal red cells within the spleen. HDFN can vary in severity from IgG sensitization of fetal red cells without apparent hemolysis to hydropic death in utero caused by severe anemia. IgM antibodies (eg, anti-I, anti-Le^a, and anti-P$_1$) do not cause HDFN because, unlike IgG, they cannot cross the placenta.

The most common cause of clinically significant HDFN is antibody to the D antigen. The incidence of Rh HDFN has declined from 13% to 0.04%,[32] primarily as a result of the use of Rh Immune Globulin (RhIG). The administration of this hyperimmune globulin prevents Rh(D) immunization in pregnant women who are D-negative. ABO incompatibility between mother and fetus can also lead to HDFN, although it is seldom clinically significant.[31] Many other blood group antigens, such as Kell, Duffy, and other Rh system antigens, can also cause maternal alloimmunization and HDFN. Antibodies against Kell antigen have been associated with severe reticulocytopenic HDFN and mild thrombocytopenia due to hemolysis and suppression of fetal hematopoiesis. As a consequence, some European countries screen for potential K1 alloimmunization.[33]

The goals of antibody screening in obstetric patients are the identification and monitoring of those females with blood group antibodies capable of causing HDFN and identification of D-negative females who should receive RhIG.[3(p43),31] Testing at an early prenatal visit should include ABO and Rh typing, as well as an antibody screen designed to detect those red cell antibodies known to cause HDFN. If the initial antibody screen is negative, a repeat antibody screen at 28 to 30 weeks of gestation should be considered in D-negative females to detect early D alloimmunization.[31,32,34] A 300-μg dose of prophylactic RhIG is administered at this time to all D-negative females. After delivery, all nonalloimmunized D-negative mothers of Rh-positive infants must receive a second dose of at least 300 μg of RhIG within 72 hours of birth. A test should be performed to assess whether excessive fetomaternal hemorrhage has occurred, in order to determine if additional RhIG must be administered to prevent D immunization.[31,32,34] (See Rh Immune Globulin in Chapter 2.)

Once it has been ascertained that a mother has become alloimmunized, the management of the pregnancy is guided by laboratory testing and ultrasound. When an antibody that is associated with HDFN is identified, an antibody titration is performed and repeated at regular intervals. If a "critical titer" of anti-D of 16 or higher is reached, the risk of fetal hydrops after 18 to 20 weeks becomes significant, and further monitoring is indicated.[31,32,34] This can include amniocentesis, middle cerebral artery peak systolic velocity (MCA-PSV) Doppler, and direct fetal blood sampling.[35]

The predictive value of titers for alloantibodies other than anti-D is uncertain, but a rising titer suggests that the fetus is at risk for HDFN and warrants more vigilant monitoring.[31] The risk of HDFN may be estimated by determining the father's red cell phenotype.[31,34] Alternatively, fetal blood type can be determined directly by DNA typing of fetal DNA in maternal plasma, amniotic fluid cells, or chorionic villi.[32,34] If fetal blood type is determined by using genetic testing, cautious interpretation may be necessary because of the complexity of the Rh loci, particularly among those of African ethnicity.[34]

Intrauterine Transfusion

To detect early signs of hydrops and to assess the severity of hemolysis, pregnancies complicated by HDFN have traditionally been monitored by serial measurements of amniotic fluid bilirubin via amniocentesis. This has largely been replaced by MCA-PSV Doppler ultrasound, a highly accurate, noninvasive method for diagnosing and monitoring the severity of anemia, as well as the fetal response to transfusion therapy.[32,34]

When severe HDFN is suspected and the fetus cannot be delivered safely, more invasive procedures are necessary. Percutaneous umbilical blood sampling (PUBS) permits antenatal blood typing, precise monitoring of fetal hematocrit, and/or direct intravascular transfusion (IVT) of the fetus. However, the rate of fetal loss from a PUBS procedure is 1% to 2%, and the procedure is not performed unless necessary.[34] A severely affected fetus may receive blood either by IVT or, much less commonly, by intraperitoneal transfusion (IPT) at periodic intervals until assessment of fetal viability indicates sufficient maturity for delivery.

Intrauterine transfusion is generally recommended when the fetal hematocrit decreases below 30%, but it is rarely feasible before 20 weeks of gestation. The volume transfused is determined according to the gestational age, estimated fetal blood volume, and the technique to be used for transfusion. The transfusion is administered via cannulation of the umbilical vein under ultrasound guidance, and it generally achieves a 10% increase in hematocrit.[34-36] The goal of transfusion is a fetal hematocrit of 25% to 50% but this endpoint should not exceed more than a fourfold increase in pretransfusion hematocrit to avoid unfavorable viscosity changes in profoundly anemic fetuses. The hematocrit is expected to decline about 1% per day, and additional IVT procedures are performed to maintain a fetal hematocrit of 40% to 50%. This usually requires IVT every 2 weeks initially and tapering to every 3 to 4 weeks after suppression of erythropoiesis.[35] Transfusions are continued until the infant is viable for delivery.[34]

RBCs for transfusion should be crossmatch compatible with the mother's serum.[3(p36)34,37] The units selected are typically group O, D-negative, hemoglobin S-negative RBCs that lack the antigen corresponding to the maternal antibody. Fresh blood, usually less than 1 week old, is preferred to ensure maximum red cell viability and to avoid low pH, decreased red cell 2,3-diphosphoglycerate (2,3-DPG), and high plasma potassium levels. The hematocrit of the RBC unit should generally be 75% to 85% to decrease the risk of volume overload in the fetus. RBCs should be irradiated to prevent GVHD, and leukocyte reduced or cytomegalovirus (CMV) seronegative for prevention of CMV transmission.[35,37]

Neonatal Transfusion Practices

Exchange Transfusion

Infants with severe hemolysis may require exchange transfusion. This technique corrects anemia and removes both antibody and potentially dangerous concentrations of bilirubin. A two-volume exchange will remove 85% of red cells and lower bilirubin by 25% to 45%.[38] Reconstituted whole blood (ie, RBCs reconstituted with group AB plasma from a different donor) is most commonly used for exchange transfusion with a final hematocrit of around 50% to 60%. The latter should result in a posttransfusion hemoglobin level of >12 g/dL.[39]

Red cells for exchange transfusion should be compatible with the mother's serum and ABO compatible with the infant. Blood less than 7 days old is usually used to ensure maximum red cell viability and to avoid decreased 2,3-DPG and high potassium levels. If fresh red cells are unavailable, older cells can be washed. As with intrauterine transfusion, red cells should be hemoglobin S-negative, leukocyte reduced or selected from

CMV-seronegative donors, and irradiated to prevent TA-GVHD.[37]

Cytomegalovirus Infection

Perinatal infection with CMV, although quite variable in its manifestations, can lead to significant morbidity and mortality. Premature infants, born to mothers who are CMV seronegative or of unknown serologic status, who weigh less than 1200 g at birth have an increased risk of transfusion-transmitted CMV. Accordingly, it is prudent to transfuse cellular blood components that have been leukocyte reduced or selected from CMV-seronegative donors to reduce the risk of CMV transmission[37,40] (see Red Blood Cells Leukocytes Reduced in Chapter 1). Some authorities recommend leukocyte-reduced or CMV-seronegative components for all children under the age of 1 year.[39]

Transfusion-Associated Graft-vs-Host Disease

TA-GVHD can occur after transfusion of immunologically competent donor lymphocytes to an immunocompromised recipient. Patients at potential risk for TA-GVHD include those with inherited or acquired defects in cellular immunity and transfusion of blood from HLA-homozygous donors. TA-GVHD is associated with intrauterine and exchange transfusion, low birthweight premature neonates, congenital defects in cellular immunity (eg, DiGeorge syndrome), fludarabine administration, immunosuppression as a result of chemotherapy or radiation therapy, HLA-matched platelets, and directed donations from first- and second-degree relatives.[3(p38),10] Irradiation of cellular blood components (RBC, platelets) is effective in preventing TA-GVHD (see Chapter 5: Adverse Effects of Blood Transfusion).

Neonatal Thrombocytopenia

Approximately 1% of newborns are thrombocytopenic at birth.[41] Severe thrombocytopenia can be the consequence of congenital infections, congenital heart disease, sepsis and disseminated intravascular coagulation (DIC), chromosomal abnormalities, maternal immune thrombocytopenia (ITP), and neonatal alloimmune thrombocytopenia (NAIT). Both maternal ITP and NAIT are caused by the passive transfer of maternal antibodies that react against the infant's platelets. NAIT occurs in approximately 1 in 1200 live births and is an important cause of isolated postnatal thrombocytopenia in an otherwise healthy term infant.[41] Analogous to HDFN and red cells, NAIT is the result of maternal antibodies directed against platelet antigens on fetal platelets, particularly HPA-1a (Pl^{A1}). Whereas maternal ITP typically runs a benign course in the infant, NAIT frequently affects the first-born infant and can cause serious intracranial hemorrhage, even before delivery. This condition may be treated in utero by the administration of intravenous gammaglobulin (IVIG) to the mother. Fetal blood sampling and direct IVT of compatible platelets (washed or plasma-reduced, irradiated, maternal platelets) is no longer recommended due to the high incidence (6%) of serious complications.

It may also be necessary to transfuse platelets and IVIG after birth. Selected platelets should be antigen-negative, if possible.[41] If antigen-negative platelets are not available, whole-blood-derived or apheresis platelets are usually efficacious.

Transfusion in Neonatal Patients

Two types of anemia develop in premature infants—iatrogenic and physiologic. In critically ill neonates, iatrogenic blood losses from repeated blood sampling required for laboratory monitoring can reach 5% of the total blood volume per day and are a major factor driving transfusion.[42] Physiologic anemia or anemia of prematurity develops a few weeks after birth and represents a physiologic decline in hemoglobin concentration. Anemia of prematurity is caused by both inadequate production and decreased responsiveness to endogenous EPO, reduced red cell lifespan, and a hyporegenerative marrow.[42] As a consequence, recombinant human EPO (rHuEPO) has only modest effects in neonates and does not reduce transfusion requirements or decrease morbidity in sick neonates.[39,40,42] In premature infants, rHuEPO may increase the rate of severe retinopathy of prematurity.[42]

The indications for transfusion in the neonate differ from those in the adult because of the infant's physiologic immaturity, small blood volume, and inability to tolerate procedure-related stress. The decision to transfuse must not be made on the basis of hemoglobin concentration alone, but rather on the basis of multiple factors, including calculated blood loss (generally 5% to 10% of total blood volume) over time, expected hemoglobin levels, reticulocyte count, and clinical status (eg, dyspnea, apnea, pallor, and poor weight gain).[40,43] There are conflicting data, however, on the usefulness of clinical signs (eg, tachycardia, tachypnea, and apnea) in an assessment of the need for RBC transfusions in the premature infant.[42] The transfusion of 10 mL/kg of RBCs over a 2- to 3-hour period should raise the hemoglobin concentration by approximately 2 to 3 g/dL.[37]

Neonatal transfusion practices vary greatly. RBC transfusions consist of an aliquot taken from a fresh blood unit. However, even from older units, the amount of potassium infused in a small-volume transfusion is clinically insignificant if the blood is transfused over a 2-hour period at a steady rate.[40,43] Washed units can be used in susceptible patients to minimize the potassium content. Red cells collected in either CPDA-1 or in additive solutions can be used safely for routine simple transfusions up to 20 mL/kg.[40,43] For rapid large-volume transfusion (eg, surgery), RBCs <7 days of age or washed RBCs are recommended. In the future, potassium adsorption filters may be available.[44]

Recent data suggest that red cells in additive solution may also be used for larger-volume transfusions.[40,45] To minimize donor exposures in an infant likely to require several transfusions, some institutions will assign a specific RBC unit to that infant. A sterile connection device is used to withdraw sequential blood aliquots for small-volume transfusions from the same unit until its outdate.[46] This protocol is applicable only to those routine transfusions that can be given slowly (2 hours) by infusion pump and not for massive or exchange transfusions.

Infants less than 4 months old rarely produce antibodies to blood group antigens; therefore, standards for pretransfusion serologic testing of these patients are different from those for testing of older infants, children, and adults.[3(pp36-37)] A pretransfusion ABO and Rh typing and an antibody screen must be performed. For neonates, maternal serum can be used for the antibody screening because any antibodies present in the infant are passively transferred from mother to infant during gestation.[31] If a clinically significant antibody is present in either maternal or fetal serum, RBC units lacking the corresponding antigen should be prepared for transfusion until the antibody is no longer identified in the infant's serum. If the initial antibody screen is negative, however, additional testing (eg, crossmatch) can be omitted provided that 1) RBCs are group O or ABO-identical or -compatible with both the mother and child and 2) RBCs are either D-negative or the same D-antigen type as the infant. Repeat testing may be omitted for infants less than 4 months of age during any one hospital admission as long as they are receiving only group O cells.[3(p27)]

In general, the primary use of plasma is in the treatment of coagulation disorders. Its use is not recommended to treat hypovolemia only. Caution should be used in interpreting coagulation studies in polycythemic samples because of excess citrate:plasma ratios in these samples.[39] As with adults, a dose of 10 to 15 mL/kg is recommended.[37,39] Plasma should be either group AB or ABO-compatible with the recipient.

Platelet transfusion practices are variable and include establishing the platelet level at which prophylactic transfusions are given to sick premature infants.[37, 39] In stable term infants, bleeding is unlikely to occur at a platelet count of 20,000/μL. In sick premature infants, a platelet count >50,000 to 100,000/μL may be needed to decrease the risk of intraventricular hemorrhage. Platelets prepared for transfusion should be ABO-identical or plasma-compatible with the patient. In an infant with NAIT, platelets should be compatible with maternal serum if possible (see later discussion). A dose of 5 to 10 mL/kg is sufficient to increase the platelet count by 50,000 to 100,000/μL.

Granulocyte transfusions have been used in some institutions for septic and neutropenic patients. The efficacy of granulocyte transfusions vs granulocyte colony-stimulating factor in septic and neutropenic neonates is still not fully established.[47]

Pediatric Transfusion Practice

Transfusion in Older Infants and Children

The clinical decision to transfuse RBCs or other blood components to older infants and children is based on the same indications as adults. Differences in blood volume, the ability to tolerate blood loss, and the normal hemoglobin and hematocrit levels for the age group in question are taken into consideration. Randomized studies have shown that stable, critically ill children can tolerate a hemoglobin level of 7 g/dL without an increase in morbidity or mortality.[48]

Sickle Cell Disease and Related Disorders

In certain chronic congenital anemias, RBC transfusions are used to suppress endogenous hemoglobin production. Children with thalassemia syndromes are given routine RBC transfusions to prevent tissue hypoxia and to suppress endogenous erythropoiesis so as to support more normal growth and development. Likewise, children with sickle cell disease who are at increased risk for a cerebrovascular accident, or who have undergone major splenic sequestration and are not candidates for splenectomy, also require chronic RBC transfusion to lower and suppress the concentration of circulating Hb S red cells.[49,50] Periodic erythrocytapheresis in sickle cell patients who have had a stroke has been effective in minimizing transfusion-related iron overload and prevention of cerebrovascular accidents.[50]

Because chronically transfused patients have a high rate of red cell alloimmunization, it is prudent to perform extended red cell phenotyping (including Rh, K, Jk, Fy, Ss) before the first transfusion in such patients.[51] In an effort to prevent red cell antibody formation and repeated delayed hemolytic reactions, many facilities use the extended red cell phenotype to administer partially matched red cells (Rh, K).[49,51] Leukocyte-reduced blood components should be used in chronically transfused patients.[49] These patients generally do not require irradiated components.

Management of Platelet Alloimmunization

Patients who repeatedly fail to achieve a therapeutic increment in platelet count after platelet transfusion are said to be refractory. The posttransfusion platelet count increment can be calculated and used to confirm the development of the refractory state (see Platelets in Chapter 1).[52] The onset of refractoriness may be associated with difficulty in controlling clinical bleeding or repeated febrile reactions to platelet transfusion. In most patients, refractoriness results from nonimmune causes such as infection, fever, DIC, active bleeding, veno-occlusive disease, and GVHD.[52] In some patients, refractoriness may be caused by the development of alloantibodies directed against foreign HLA and/or platelet-specific antigens.

The most common alloantibodies associated with platelet refractoriness are directed against Class I antigens in the HLA system. These antigens are expressed on platelets and all nucleated cells. HLA antibodies develop after exposure to foreign HLA antigens, as may occur during pregnancy, after the transfusion of cellular blood components, and organ transplantation. Less commonly, patients become refractory because of platelet-specific (non-HLA) antibodies, ABO incompatibility, or drug-induced antibodies. The possibility of ITP or posttransfusion purpura should also be considered. The diagnosis of alloimmunization is supported by a positive test for antibodies to HLA antigens or by a positive platelet crossmatch.

Effective therapies for alloimmunized patients with severe thrombocytopenia are limited.[52] Platelet transfusions from HLA-unmatched donors are nearly always ineffective, but the use of platelets from HLA-matched donors or family members may restore platelet responsiveness. The extensive polymorphism of the HLA system, however, can preclude the procurement of sufficient HLA-identical donors to meet the needs of refractory patients. The transfusion of platelets from partially or selectively HLA-matched donors may be successful if the match is close enough. Another method for selecting compatible donors compares HLA amino acid sequence information between donor and recipient. Identifying the specificity of the HLA antibody (a process that is analogous to red cell antibody identification) may permit a wider choice of donors with known HLA types.

Platelet crossmatching, in which patient serum/plasma is tested against a panel of single-donor platelets, has also been successful. Platelet crossmatching can be extremely helpful when patients do not have an HLA type on record or there are significant delays in scheduling and obtaining HLA-selected platelets. In addition, direct platelet crossmatching can detect incompatibilities to both HLA and platelet-specific antibodies.[51] Platelet crossmatching is limited by the amount of serum/plasma available for testing.

In some cases, even the use of well-matched platelets does not result in an adequate posttransfusion increment. This may result from the presence of complicating nonimmune factors or to platelet ABO incompatibility. Other approaches to clinically managing platelet refractoriness, such as the use of high-dose IVIG, plasmapheresis, splenectomy, or epsilon-aminocaproic acid, have met with marginal success.[52]

Evidence indicates that platelets themselves are not highly immunogenic and that passenger leukocytes in the transfusion product are responsible for the induction of platelet antibodies. Leukocyte reduction has been shown to significantly reduce the incidence of primary HLA alloimmunization.[53] Leukocyte reduction does not prevent the secondary immune resurgence of existing HLA antibodies in patients who were previously immunized through pregnancy or transfusion.

Administration of Blood

The most common cause of fatal hemolytic transfusion reactions is the misidentification of either the blood unit or the recipient.[10] Among the steps that are necessary for safe transfusion, the positive identification of the patient and the blood sample are the most critical. After sample collection, identification systems must be in place to ensure that technical and clerical errors are not made.

At the time of transfusion, the blood component with the compatibility tag attached (this tag should not be removed) must be compared with the patient's identification bracelet. No discrepancies in spelling or identification numbers should exist. The patient should remain under close observation for 15 minutes after the infusion begins and must be assessed periodically until an appropriate time after the transfusion is completed.[3(p42),54] In a stable adult, blood components are usually administered over 30 (plasma, platelets) to 120 minutes (RBCs). Blood may be given more slowly in patients who are sensitive to fluid imbalances. As a general rule in stable pediatric patients, blood components are administered at 10 mL/kg over 2 to 3 hours. Infusion rate is dependent on adequate venous access and needle size. For adults, a 20-to 18-gauge needle is appropriate for routine transfusion. In infants and toddlers, the smallest gauge for RBC infusion is 24-to 22-gauge and will require a syringe and pump for administration.[54]

Time Limits for Infusing Blood Components

A unit of RBCs should not be kept at room temperature for more than a short time because of the risk of bacterial growth. Blood should be infused within 4 hours. If that time is likely to be exceeded, the unit should be divided into aliquots using a sterile connection device, and portions kept in the blood bank refrigerator until required. A unit of blood that has been allowed to warm above 10 C, but is not used, cannot be reissued by the transfusion service. Blood must never be stored in unmonitored refrigerators.

Blood Warming

Transfusion of cold blood at more than 100 mL/minute has been associated with a higher rate of cardiac arrest than transfusion of warmed blood in a control group.[55] At routine flow rates—ie, those slower than 100 mL/minute—transfused blood does not require warming, because the patient's body heat quickly warms each drop to equilibrium as the blood enters the vein. Unless a severe cold autoimmune hemolytic anemia is present, blood warming is not usually required. In the trauma setting, rapid infusion devices are often integral to blood-warming devices, and they come as a combined instrument. These instruments can rapidly warm and infuse the blood either through peripheral IV catheters of 14- to 18-gauge or central IV catheters of larger diameter. Most infusion devices have special disposable kits with larger-gauge tubing that are specifically designed for use with the device. Warming devices mostly use dry heat, but they can also use waterbaths, countercurrent heat exchange, or in-line microwave technology. Modern warmers typically have sensors to tightly compensate for changes in blood flow and to maintain equal warming of blood and other infusibles. Automatic warming devices must have a visible thermometer and should have an audible warning system. Warming the whole unit of blood by immersion in hot water or by the use of microwave blood warmers is contraindicated because hemolysis can result from overheating.

The use of blood warmers is generally restricted to rapid and multiple transfusions to adult patients at more than 50 mL/minute for 30 minutes or more, to the patient rewarming phase of cardiopulmonary bypass surgery, to exchange transfusions in infants, to transfusions to children in volumes greater than 15 mL/kg/hour, and in cases of severe cold autoimmune hemolytic anemia.

Infusion Devices

Several electronic infusion devices (ie, blood pumps) are available. These machines are designed to deliver parenteral fluids, including blood components, at flow rates ranging from 1 mL/minute to more than 1 L/minute. The pump mechanisms vary with different manufacturers and include syringe-type pumping systems, peristaltic roller devices, and electromechanical pumps that operate on a positive volumetric displacement principle. Rapid infusion systems can be as simple as an inflatable cuff with a pocket and sphygmomanometer or can include electronic instruments that more tightly control the pressure and flow rates. Electronic rapid infusion devices will monitor pressure and compensate to maintain the desired flow without exceeding 300 mm Hg pressure to the bag. Some systems require manufacturer-supplied pump cassettes, whereas others can be used with standard IV administration set tubing. Although most pump systems do not induce mechanical hemolysis when used with Whole Blood, gross hemolysis can result when some models are used to administer RBCs. The manufacturer's insert should be consulted for approval for use with blood components. Peak infusion rates and the degree of hemolysis depend on both the infusion device and the sizes of tubing and catheter used.[56,57]

Concomitant Use of Intravenous Solutions

Only normal saline (0.9% USP) may be administered with blood components. Other solutions may be hypotonic (eg, 5% dextrose in water) and may cause hemolysis in vitro, or they may contain additives such as calcium (lactated Ringer's solution) that can initiate in-vitro coagulation in citrated blood.[58] However, despite some studies showing no increase in coagulation with lactated Ringer's solution, normal saline remains the only acceptable solution for mixing with blood components.[59] RBCs may be diluted with normal saline to decrease viscosity and increase the infusion rate. Medications should never be added to a unit of blood or infused with blood. Some drugs may cause hemolysis because of their excessively high pH. Furthermore, if medication is added to blood and the transfusion is discontinued for any reason, the dose of infused medication may not be known. Finally, it would be difficult to determine whether any adverse transfusion reactions were caused by the blood or the drug it contained.

Filters

All blood components must be administered through a filter in order to remove blood clots and other debris. Standard blood filters, with a pore size between 170 and 260 microns, trap large aggregates and clots. Microaggregate blood filters with 20- to 40-micron pores can remove microaggregate debris, and they are frequently employed when blood is recirculated in cardiac bypass devices. They are not indicated for routine blood transfusions and do not accomplish leukocyte reduction. Blood filters designed for leukocyte-reduced cellular blood components are available (see Red Blood Cells Leukocytes Reduced in Chapter 1). Disadvantages of both microaggregate and leukocyte reduction filters include the potential to become clogged and resistance to rapid blood delivery. These problems may be circumvented by using components that have been leukocyte reduced by the blood donor center before issue.

References

1. Palmer T, Wahr JA, O'Reilly M, Greenfield ML. Reducing unnecessary cross-matching: A patient-specific blood

ordering system is more accurate in predicting who will receive a blood transfusion than the maximum blood ordering system. Anesth Analg 2003;96:369-75.

2. Friedman BA, Oberman HA, Chadwick AR, Kingdon KI. The maximum surgical blood order schedule and surgical blood use in the United States. Transfusion 1976;16:380-7.

3. Carson TH, ed. Standards for blood banks and transfusion services. 27th ed. Bethesda, MD: AABB, 2011.

4. Butch SH, Oberman HA. The computer or electronic crossmatch. Transfus Med Rev 1997;11:256-64.

5. Padget BJ, Hannon JL. Variations in pretransfusion practices. Immunohematology 2003;19:1-6.

6. Waters JH, ed. Blood management: Options for better patient care. Bethesda, MD: AABB Press, 2008.

7. Ferraris VA, Ferraris SP, Saha SP et al. Perioperative blood transfusion and blood conservation in cardiac surgery: The society of thoracic surgeons and the society of cardiovascular anesthesiologists clinical practice guidelines. Ann Thorac Surg 2007;83:S27-86.

8. Ilstrup S, ed. Standards for perioperative autologous blood collection and administration. 4th ed. Bethesda, MD: AABB, 2009.

9. Waters JH, Dyga RM, Yazer MH. Guidelines for blood recovery and reinfusion in surgery and trauma. Bethseda, MD: AABB, 2010.

10. Popovsky MA, ed. Transfusion reactions. 3rd ed. Bethesda, MD: AABB Press, 2007.

11. Tasaki T, Ohto H. Nineteen years of experience with autotransfusion for elective surgery in children: More troublesome than we expected. Transfusion 2007;47:1503-9.

12. Popovsky MA, Whitaker B, Arnold NL. Severe outcomes of allogeneic and autologous blood donation: Frequency and characterization. Transfusion 1995;35:734-7.

13. Silvergleid AJ. Safety and effectiveness of predeposit autologous transfusions in preteen and adolescent children. JAMA 1987;257:3403-4.

14. Carless PA, Henry DA, Moxey AJ, et al. Cell salvage for minimizing perioperative allogeneic blood transfusion. Cochrane Database Syst Rev 2010;(4):CD001888.

15. Hansen E, Pawlik M. Reasons against the retransfusion of unwashed wound blood. Transfusion 2004;44(Suppl):45S-53S.

16. Stramer SL, Glynn SA, Kleinman SH, et al. Detection of HIV-1 and HCV infections among antibody-negative blood donors by nucleic acid-amplification testing. N Engl J Med 2004;351:760-8.

17. Oberman HA, Barnes BA, Friedman BA. The risk of abbreviating the major crossmatch in urgent or massive transfusion. Transfusion 1978;18:137-41.

18. Brohi K, Cohen MJ, Davenport RA. Acute coagulopathy of trauma: Mechanism, identification and effect. Curr Opin Crit Care 2007;13:680-5.

19. Frith D, Brohi K. The acute coagulopathy of trauma shock: Clinical relevance. Surgeon 2010:8:159-163.

20. Kashuk JL, Moore EE, Johnson JL, et al. Postinjury life threatening coagulopathy: Is 1:1 fresh frozen plasma: Packed red blood cells the answer? J Trauma 2008:65:261-71.

21. Perry DJ, Fizmaurice DA, Kitchen S, et al. Point-of-care testing in haemostasis. Br J Haematol 2010;150:501-14.

22. Shackford SR, Virgilio RW, Peters RM. Whole blood versus packed-cell transfusions: A physiologic comparison. Ann Surg 1981;193:337-40.

23. Mannucci PM, Levi M. Prevention and treatment of major blood loss. N Engl J Med 2007;356:2301-11.

24. Ciavarella D, Reed RL, Counts RB, et al. Clotting factor levels and the risk of diffuse microvascular bleeding in the massively transfused patient. Br J Haematol 1987;67:365-8.

25. Ramsey G, Sherman LA. Transfusion therapy in solid organ transplantation. Hematol Oncol Clin North Am 1994;8:1117-29.

26. Wegner JA, DiNardo JA, Arabia FA, Copeland JG. Blood loss and transfusion requirements in patients implanted

with a mechanical support device undergoing cardiac transplantation. J Heart Lung Transplant 2000;19:504-6.

27. Wu A, Buhler LH, Cooper DKC. ABO-incompatible organ and bone marrow transplantation: Current status. Transpl Int 2003;16:291-9.

28. West LJ, Pollock-Barziv SM, Dipchand AI, et al. ABO-incompatible heart transplantation in infants. N Engl J Med 2001;344:793-800.

29. Oyelese Y, Ananth CV. Postpartum hemorrhage: Epidemiology, risk factors and causes. Clin Obstet Gynecol 2010; 53:147-56

30. Rajan PV, Wing DA. Postpartum hemorrhage: Evidence-based medical interventions for prevention and treatment. Clin Obstet Gynecol 2010;53:165-81.

31. Judd WJ, for the Scientific Section Coordinating Committee. Guidelines for prenatal and perinatal immunohematology. Bethesda, MD: AABB, 2005.

32. Liumbruno GM, D'Alessandro A, Rea F, et al. The role of antenatal immunoprophylaxis in the prevention of maternal-foetal anti-Rh(D) alloimmunization. Blood Transfus 2010;8:8-16.

33. Schonewille H, Klumper FJCM, van de Watering LMG. High additional maternal red cell alloimmunization after Rhesus- and K-matched intrauterine intravascular transfusions for hemolytic disease of the fetus. Am J Obstet Gynecol 2007;196:143e1-e6.

34. Moise KJ Jr. Management of rhesus alloimmunization in pregnancy. Obstet Gynecol 2008;112:164-76.

35. Oepkes D, Adama va Scheltema P. Intrauterine fetal transfusions in the management of fetal anemia and fetal thrombocytopenia. Semin Fetal Neonatal Med 2007;12:432-8.

36. Giannina G, Moise KJ Jr, Dorman K. A simple method to estimate volume for fetal intravascular transfusions. Fetal Diagn Ther 1998;13:94-7.

37. Wu Y, Stack G. Blood product replacement in the perinatal period. Semin Perinatal 2007;31:262-71.

38. American Academy of Pediatrics Subcommittee on Hyper-bilirubinemia, Clinical Practice Guidelines: Management of hyperbilirubinemia in the newborn infant 35 or more weeks in gestation. Pediatrics 2004;114:297-316.

39. British Committee for Standards in Haematology. Transfusion guidelines for neonates and older children. Br J Haematol 2004;124:433-53.

40. Strauss RG. Data-driven blood banking practices for neonatal RBC transfusions. Transfusion 2000;40:1528-40.

41. Crowley M, Kirpalani H. A rational approach to red blood cell transfusion in the neonatal ICU. Curr Opin Pediatr 2010;22:151-7.

42. Strauss RG. Red blood cell transfusion and avoiding hyperkalemia to neonates and infants. Transfusion 2010;50:1862-65.

43. Yamada C, Heitmiller ES, Ness PM, King KE. Reduction in potassium concentration of stored red blood cell units using a resin filter. Transfusion 2010;50:1926-33.

44. Mou SS, Giroir BP, Molitor-Kirsch EA, et al. Fresh whole blood versus reconstituted blood for pump priming in heart surgery in infants. N Engl J Med 2004;351:1635-44.

45. Liu EA, Mannino FL, Lane TA. Prospective, randomized trial of the safety and efficacy of a limited donor exposure transfusion program for premature neonates. J Pediatr 1994;125:92-6.

46. Mohan P, Brocklehurst P. Granulocyte transfusions for neonates with confirmed or suspected sepsis and neutropaenia. Cochrane Database Syst Rev 2003;(4):CD003956.

47. Lacroix J, Hebert PC, Hutchison JS, et al. Transfusion strategies for patients in pediatric intensive care units. N Engl J Med 2007;356:1609-19.

48. Roseff SD. Sickle cell disease: A review. Immunohematology 2009;25:67-74.

49. Lee MT, Piomelli S, Granger S, et al. Stroke prevention trial in sickle cell anemia (STOP): Extended follow-up and final results. Blood 2006;108:847-52.

50. Vichinsky EP, Luban NL, Wright E, et al. Prospective RBC phenotype matching in a stroke-prevention trial in sickle cell anemia: A multicenter transfusion trial. Transfusion 2001;41:1086-92.

51. Arnold DM, Sith JW, Kelton JG. Diagnosis and management of neonatal alloimmune thrombocytopenia. Transfus Med Rev 2008;22:255-67.

52. Hod E, Schwartz J. Platelet transfusion refractoriness. Br J Haematol 2008;142:348-60.

53. Leukocyte reduction and ultraviolet B irradiation of platelets to prevent alloimmunization and refractoriness to platelet transfusions. The Trial to Reduce Alloimmunization to Platelets Study Group. N Engl J Med 1997;337:1861-9.

54. Sink B. Adminstration of blood components. In: Roback JD, Grossman, BJ, Harris T, Hillyer C, eds. Technical manual. 17th ed. Bethesda, MD: AABB, 2011:613-24.

55. Boyan CP, Howland WS. Cardiac arrest and temperature of bank blood. JAMA 1963;183:58-60.

56. Frelich R, Ellis MH. The effect of external pressure, catheter gauge, and storage time on hemolysis in RBC transfusion. Transfusion 2001;41:799-802.

57. Millikan JS, Cain TL, Hansbrough J. Rapid volume replacement for hypovolemic shock: A comparison of techniques and equipment. J Trauma 1984;24:428-31.

58. Ryden SE, Oberman HA. Compatibility of common intravenous solutions with CPD blood. Transfusion 1975;15:250-5.

59. Lorenzo M, Davis JW, Negin S, et al. Can Ringer's lactate be used safely with blood transfusions? Am J Surg 1998;175:308-10.

HEMOSTATIC DISORDERS

Overview of Hemostasis

Hemostasis refers to the physiologic mechanisms that control bleeding. Normal hemostasis may be viewed as occurring in three overlapping stages. Primary hemostasis involves blood vessels (particularly the endothelial layer) and cellular blood elements (particularly platelets) and culminates in the formation of the platelet plug. The second stage of hemostasis involves plasma procoagulant proteins (clotting or coagulation factors) and the formation of a stable fibrin clot. The third stage involves repair of vascular damage that results in a return to the normal state. Two control processes, the fibrinolytic system and an anticoagulant system (consisting of inhibitor proteins and endothelial-cell-based mechanisms), are important in limiting clot formation to areas of vascular injury. Pathologic bleeding or thrombosis may result from derangement in any of these processes.

Blood Vessels

Under conditions of normal health, vascular endothelium maintains a thromboresistant surface by a variety of mechanisms, including secretion of the platelet inhibitory substances (such as prostacyclin and nitric oxide), expression of molecules involved in the inhibition of coagulation (eg, heparan and thrombomodulin), and provision of a barrier between intravascular elements and the tissue factor (TF)-rich extravascular structures. After injury, the blood vessel constricts, which limits blood flow. The interaction of blood elements with subendothelial structures allows adhesion and activation of platelets, and activation of pro-coagulant mechanisms. Within minutes fibrin formation occurs, which results in a stable platelet-fibrin clot.

Hereditary blood vessel disorders associated with a bleeding diathesis include connective tissue disorders (eg, Ehlers-Danlos and Marfan syndromes) and vascular malformations (eg, heredi-tary hemorrhagic telangiectasia syndrome and giant hemangioma).

Acquired blood vessel disorders include medical conditions such as scurvy and vasculitis, vascular anomalies such as angiod-ysplasia, and physical disruptions such as occurs with trauma or surgery. If available, treatment is directed to the underlying vas-cular abnormality. Postoperative anatomic bleeding caused by inadequate surgical hemostasis may be difficult to diagnose, par-ticularly in patients with concomitant abnormalities of platelets or coagulation factors. In general, bleeding from one site sug-gests an anatomical lesion, whereas small-vessel bleeding from multiple sites (eg, wound edges, intravenous access sites, and the endotracheal tube) suggests abnormal hemostatic mechanisms.

Platelets

Platelets are anuclear cell fragments that form a cohesive plug at the site of vessel injury. Both thrombocytopenia and platelet function defects are causes of abnormal hemostasis. The platelet component of hemostasis is routinely assessed by two screening methods: the platelet count and platelet function assessment. In patients who are actively bleeding or who are about to undergo major invasive procedures, platelet transfusions are often indi-cated for counts below 50,000/µL.[1-3] Higher counts may be desired for procedures in which any increased bleeding would be problematic, such as neurologic, thoracic, or ophthalmologic sur-gery.[4] In nonbleeding patients with thrombocytopenia caused by marrow failure, prophylactic platelet transfusions are generally reserved for platelet counts below 10,000/µL.[2] However, there is some evidence that using a lower transfusion threshold or withholding transfusion unless bleeding is evident may also be safe strategies.[1] Although clinical factors such as fever, sepsis, splenomegaly, renal failure, or drugs (eg, amphotericin) have been used to justify a higher threshold (ie, 20,000/μL), the effectiveness of that strategy has been questioned.[2] Response to prophylactic platelet transfusion should be assessed to help guide continued therapy and to detect platelet refractoriness (see Chapter 1: Blood Components and Chapter 3: Transfusion Practices).[1]

Evaluation of platelet hemostatic function in a patient with a history of bleeding symptoms remains difficult.[5] The template bleeding time may be prolonged in patients with von Willebrand disease (VWD) and platelet function defects, but this test has been eliminated at most centers owing to its poor diagnostic accuracy and its lack of prognostic value as a predictor of surgical bleeding.[6] The platelet function analyzer (PFA-100, Siemens, Deerfield, IL) closure time is an alternative to the bleeding time; the result reported is the time required for platelets and plasma proteins in a patient's whole-blood sample to generate an obstructive aggregate at the aperture of a collagen-coated membrane.[6] The PFA-100 assay detects relatively severe defects including abnormalities of platelet adhesion (eg, VWD or Bernard-Soulier syndrome), abnormalities of platelet secretion (eg, storage pool defect, aspirin effect, etc) and disorders of aggregation (eg, Glanzmann thrombasthenia). Cohort studies suggest that the PFA-100 assay is less informative for detection of milder forms of VWD and less-well-defined platelet function defects.[6] A patient with a significant history of bleeding in the face of an adequate platelet count merits evaluation of von Willebrand factor (VWF) and/or platelet aggregation studies. Finally, it is worth noting that the PFA-100 assay lacks the sensitivity or specificity to be used as a routine preoperative screening tool, and does not replace a detailed clinical history in predicting the risk of surgical bleeding.[6]

Platelets play an important role in the coagulation system as well. Coagulation proteins and Ca^{++} are stored within platelet granules, and coagulation factors assemble on the phospholipid surface of activated platelets. Aspirin is a mild platelet antagonist that inhibits platelet thromboxane production, whereas thienopyridines (eg, clopidogrel and prasugrel) inhibit the platelet adenosine diphosphate (ADP) receptor. Aspirin and clopidogrel are irreversible inhibitors of platelet function. Recommendations for delaying surgery for patients taking these agents varies depending upon the indications for which the medications are being administered, the surgical bleeding risk, and the interval between surgery and the patient's last dose of medication.[4] Glycoprotein (GP) IIb-IIIa inhibitors (eg, abciximab, eptifibatide, and tirofiban) are potent inhibitors of platelet aggregation that block the GPIIb-IIIa receptor for fibrinogen and VWF. They also inhibit thrombin generation and platelet procoagulant activity and prolong the activated clotting time. These drugs significantly reduce thrombotic complications in patients with acute coronary syndromes who are undergoing percutaneous coronary intervention.[7] Platelet function returns to about half the pretreatment status in about 4 to 12 hours depending on the drug given.[8] Patients who develop bleeding after receiving the longer acting GPIIb-IIIa inhibitor abciximab may require repeated platelet transfusions to counteract the effect of the drug. Thrombocytopenia is an infrequent complication of GPIIb-IIIa inhibitor therapy and is seen in less than 1.0% of cases.[9] Discontinuation of the GPIIb-IIIa inhibitor is recommended with thrombocytopenia, and in severe cases, platelet transfusion may be appropriate.

Coagulation Proteins

The initial platelet plug that forms at a site of vascular injury is stabilized by fibrin. The fibrin is generated by the coagulation mechanism, which consists of a closely regulated series of reactions culminating in the transformation of fibrinogen into an insoluble fibrin matrix. The coagulation mechanism consists of procoagulant serine proteases that circulate as zymogens (ie, Factors II, VII, IX, X, XI, and XII), nonenzymatic cofactors (ie, Factors V and VIII), the substrate for fibrin gel formation (fibrinogen), and fibrin-stabilizing enzymes [Factor XIII and thrombin activatable fibrinolysis inhibitor (TAFI)].

In vivo, the exposure of TF to blood is the key step in the initiation of coagulation.[10] TF is abundantly present in the subendothelium, may be expressed on activated endothelial cells (and possibly synthesized by activated platelets), and may also be transported to sites of vascular injury in the form of circulating microparticles. TF triggers the coagulation system at the site of injury by capturing circulating Factor VIIa. The Factor VIIa-TF complex converts Factor X to its active form either directly or indirectly via activation of Factor IX. Phospholipid membrane-bound Factor Xa then forms a complex with Factor Va, which in turn converts the zymogen prothrombin to the active enzyme thrombin. Thrombin dissociates from the membrane surface and converts fibrinogen to fibrin and activates Factor XIII. Factor XIIIa stabilizes the clot by covalent crosslinking of fibrin. Thrombin amplifies the coagulation signal by feedback activation of Factors XI, IX, VIII, and V. This positive feedback sustains coagulation after the Factor VIIa-TF process is inhibited by TF pathway inhibitor. Inadequate amplification of the initial hemostatic signal is thought to explain why hemophiliacs bleed despite normal levels of Factor VII.

In vitro, coagulation can be initiated by another protease/cofactor system, the so-called contact factor system. Deficiencies of the contact factors (ie, Factor XII, prekallikrein, and kininogen) will prolong the activated partial thromboplastin time (aPTT) screening test (see below) but are not associated with a clinical bleeding diathesis.

Screening of coagulation includes both clinical history and 1) the prothrombin time (PT, which evaluates the extrinsic pathway that includes Factors VII, X, V, II and fibrinogen); 2) the aPTT (which evaluates the intrinsic pathway that includes contact Factors XI, IX, VIII, X, V, II and fibrinogen); 3) the thrombin time (TT, which evaluates the fibrinogen-to-fibrin conversion step and is sensitive to the effect of heparin); and 4) a quantitative fibrinogen assay. Acquired mild-to-moderate prolongation of the PT that results from liver disease is often associated with significant decreases in coagulation factor levels or with an increased bleeding risk.[11-13] However, in congenital hemostatic disorders (such as mild hemophilia), minor abnormalities of the PT or aPTT may be indicators of a clinically significant coagulation factor deficiency. Therapeutic levels of the coagulation factors required for hemostasis and the indications for factor replacement depend upon the patient's clinical status and the magnitude of the hemostatic challenge. Coagulation factor levels above 25% to 35% and fibrinogen levels above 100 mg/dL are sufficient to prevent major hemorrhage,[14,15] but higher levels may be desirable for patients facing major surgery or with trauma-related bleeding.[4,16]

Both congenital and acquired disorders of coagulation occur. Common congenital disorders include VWD and the hemophilias, and common acquired disorders include vitamin K deficiency, liver disease, consumptive coagulopathy, dilutional coagulopathy, and medication effects.

Natural Anticoagulant Systems and Fibrinolysis

The processes by which procoagulant activities are limited to the site of injury are important regulators of normal hemostasis. Two main processes are involved: the natural anticoagulant systems, which consist primarily of circulating and endothelial-based protease inhibitors, and the fibrinolytic system, which is primarily responsible for the proteolytic dissolution of the fibrin clot. Blood fluidity depends largely on the integrity of the two anticoagulant proteins, antithrombin and protein C. Antithrombin inhibits thrombin and other activated coagulation serine proteases. Antithrombin is a weak inhibitor by itself, but heparin and heparan-like molecules markedly augment its activity. Protein C is activated by thrombin bound to thrombomodulin on endothelial cells. Activated protein C, in the presence of protein S, degrades Factors Va and VIIIa. The protein C system subserves both anticoagulant and antiapoptotic/anti-inflammatory functions. A mutation in Factor V (Factor V Leiden) results in resistance to the anticoagulant action of activated protein C and increased risk of venous thrombosis.[17]

Fibrinolysis is accomplished by the enzyme plasmin, which is formed by the action of endothelial-cell-based activators upon its circulating zymogen, plasminogen. Plasminogen activator (tissue type or urokinase type) converts plasminogen to plasmin. Plasmin binds to the newly formed fibrin and breaks it down to soluble degradation products, which leads to clot lysis. Unbound plasmin can degrade fibrinogen, Factor V, and Factor VIII. In-vivo regulation of plasmin activity occurs at two levels: 1) plasminogen activator inhibitor (PAI) blocks the activation of plasminogen by the plasminogen activators, and 2) α_2 antiplasmin inhibits plasmin. An increased level of plasminogen activator, a deficiency of PAI, or a deficiency of α_2 antiplasmin may cause a bleeding tendency through increased plasmin activity.

Conversely, derangement of the fibrinolytic mechanisms may increase thrombotic risk. Examples include increased PAI and resistance of fibrin to the normal action of plasmin in thrombotic dysfibrinogenemias. One link between fibrinolysis and coagulation is TAFI. TAFI is activated by thrombin, and it reduces the efficiency of clot lysis by plasmin. Whether elevated TAFI levels are associated with a mild risk for venous thrombosis is unclear.[18]

Laboratory markers of an activated fibrinolytic system are not readily available.[19] A shortened (<60 minute) euglobulin clot lysis time indicates a fibrinolytic state. A decrease in the plasma fibrinogen level or an elevation of TT, fibrin degradation products, or D-dimer, may also point to activated fibrinolysis. An elevation of these degradation products can inhibit fibrin formation and impair platelet function. Severe liver disease and hepatic surgery (resection or transplantation) are the most common causes of primary fibrinolysis. In surgical settings, thromboelastogram monitoring may be used to detect an early decrease in clot strength with accelerated fibrinolysis.[20]

Platelet Disorders

Many conditions can result in thrombocytopenia. When it results from marrow suppression (from radiation, chemotherapy, nutritional deficiency, or toxic drugs), platelet transfusions are usually successful in elevating the platelet count and lowering the bleeding risk. Multiple factors may result in a decreased responsiveness to platelet transfusion.[1] In addition to disease-related factors [such as splenomegaly, sepsis, fever, disseminated intravascular coagulation (DIC), or complications of hematopoietic stem cell transplantation], patients who have been repeatedly transfused or pregnant may develop antibodies to HLA or platelet-specific antigens that are present on the platelet surface. Frequently, these refractory patients will respond to transfusions of crossmatch-compatible or HLA-selected platelets. The use of ABO-compatible platelets and leukocyte-reduced blood components reduces the rate of alloimmunization and refractoriness to platelet transfusions in patients with acute leukemia.[1]

In contrast, accelerated destruction of peripheral blood platelets (because of consumptive or immune disorders) is more difficult to treat with transfusions because the transfused platelets are rapidly destroyed. For this reason, transfusion to increase the platelet count is generally not helpful in autoimmune thrombocytopenia; however, transfusion may be useful in the management of acute hemorrhage.[1,2,21] Anecdotal reports of disease exacerbation suggest that platelet transfusions are hazardous in patients with thrombotic thrombocytopenic purpura (TTP) or heparin-induced thrombocytopenia (HIT). These patients should receive platelet transfusion only when it is medically necessary for control of active bleeding.[22,23]

Platelet function defects may be congenital or acquired.[5,24] Congenital disorders include abnormalities of platelet granules or membrane receptors. Acquired disorders are most often caused by drugs, especially aspirin, nonsteroidal anti-inflammatory agents, and platelet receptor antagonists (thienopyridines and GPIIb-IIIa inhibitors). Patients with uremia and those undergoing procedures involving extracorporeal circulation may have platelet function defects.[25]

Desmopressin (DDAVP) has been reported to be effective in treating bleeding associated with both uremia and congenital platelet function abnormalities.[25] DDAVP releases Factor VIII and VWF from endothelial cells and other storage sites, but other mechanisms may also be contributing to the therapeutic effect (see Prohemostatic Drugs below for details of administration). Response to DDAVP in a patient with a platelet function defect is empirically assessed; there is no convincing evidence that laboratory monitoring is useful. Platelet transfusion can be used to treat selected platelet function defects, but the hemostatic defect seen with uremia will not respond to platelet transfusion alone. Treatment of bleeding in uremic patients without thrombocytopenia includes dialysis, maintenance of the hematocrit >30%,[24] and administration of DDAVP and conjugated estrogens. For some patients, systemic or topical administration of antifibrinolytic therapy may be appropriate. Finally, recombinant Factor VIIa has proven effective in patients with Glanzmann thrombasthenia, but this is not a licensed indication in the United States.[25]

Congenital Bleeding Disorders

von Willebrand Disease

VWD is a very common hereditary bleeding disorder,[26] which may result from quantitative or qualitative abnormalities of VWF. VWF is a large multimeric molecule that is secreted from endothelial cells, is present in both plasma and platelets, and mediates platelet adhesion to subendothelial tissues at sites of vascular injury. Platelet plug formation is defective in patients with VWD. Another VWF function is as a chaperone for coagulation Factor VIII. Diminished Factor VIII levels are frequently seen in patients with VWD. Regulation of VWF function is complex, and the metalloprotease ADAMTS13 is involved in prevention of inappropriate VWF-platelet microthrombi (see section on TTP). VWD manifests most commonly as mucosal bleeding, but deep tissue bleeding can occur in severe cases. A diagnosis of VWD is confirmed by specific assays of both VWF and Factor VIII.[26] Because of the multiplicity of VWF defects, a classification system has been adopted. The most common form of VWD is mild-to-moderate quantitative VWF deficiency (type 1 VWD). In patients in whom production of VWF is virtually absent (type 3 VWD), Factor VIII levels are in the same range as those in patients with moderate hemophilia A. Type 3 VWD is inherited as an autosomal recessive disorder, but the condition can be mimicked in rare individuals on an autoimmune basis. While types 2A, 2B, and 2M VWD are all attributable to structural defects of VWF that undermine the interaction of VWF with platelets, patients with type 2N VWD manifest unexpectedly low Factor VIII levels caused by impaired transporter function of VWF.

DDAVP is primarily useful to increase VWF levels and restore hemostatic function in patients with type 1 VWD. DDAVP is not useful in patients with severe (type 3) disease. The utility of DDAVP in the qualitative variants (types 2A, 2M, and 2N) is patient-specific and less predictable, and DDAVP is relatively contraindicated in individuals with qualitative variants characterized by increased interaction between VWF and platelets (type 2B and platelet-type VWD), as DDAVP administration may worsen thrombocytopenia in those patients. DDAVP is usually given in doses of 0.3 µg/kg intravenously over 20 minutes, but it is also available as a concentrated nasal spray. Administration of an elective test dose is helpful to confirm a patient's responsiveness, and most patients with type 1 VWD experience a twofold to fivefold increase of VWF levels 30 to 60 minutes after infusion. DDAVP-induced elevation of VWF levels persists for about 8 to 10 hours.[26]

Tachyphylaxis may develop; thus, DDAVP may not be effective after three or four consecutive daily doses.[27] Mild and transient side effects include headache and facial flushing. To prevent hyponatremia and water retention caused by the antidiuretic effect of DDAVP, patients should restrict fluid intake for 24 hours after DDAVP administration. DDAVP should be used with caution in elderly individuals with cardiovascular disease and in children weighing <20 kg. Pregnancy is not a contraindication for DDAVP; however, its use may complicate fluid management. Furthermore, many patients with type 1 VWD will experience an increase in VWF levels by the end of pregnancy sufficient that they can undergo parturition without requiring additional support of the VWF level.[26]

Patients who are unresponsive to DDAVP or have type 2B and type 3 variants require exogenous VWF-containing factor concentrate. Virus-inactivated products are recommended and, currently, Humate-P (CSL Behring, King of Prussia, PA), Alphanate (Grifols Biologicals, Los Angeles, CA), and Wilate (Octapharma, Hoboken, NJ) are plasma-derived VWF-containing concentrates that are both labeled in VWF ristocetin cofactor activity units (VWF:RCo units) and approved by the Food and Drug Administration (FDA) for the treatment of VWD. High-purity Factor VIII concentrates prepared by monoclonal or recombinant technology are devoid of VWF and should not be used for treatment of VWD. Although Cryoprecipitated Antihemophilic Factor (AHF) contains both Factor VIII and VWF, its use in the treatment of VWD (or hemophilia A) should be reserved for urgent situations when virus-attenuated factor concentrates are not immediately available. Although Cryoprecipitated AHF is not quality assured for VWF contents, reports suggest it contains approximately 90 to 170 VWF:RCo units per individual product.[28] Dose calculation of VWF-containing concentrates is performed by determining the desired increment of VWF level; administration of 1.0 VWF:RCo unit/kg will generally result in an increase in VWF activity of approximately 1.5% (ie, 0.015 IU/mL or 1.5 units/dL; see Table 4 for dose calculations). For life-threatening bleeding or major surgery, a recommended initial target VWF:RCo level of 80% to 100% is suggested, and follow-up therapy is aimed at preserving hemostatic levels for at least 3 days. However, recommendations for the duration of factor support vary widely between surgical procedures.[26] For minor bleeding episodes, a single dose chosen to achieve a VWF:RCo level of 40% to 50% may be sufficient.[26] In a patient with the type 2N VWD (in which the Factor VIII levels are lower than VWF levels because of an abnormal interaction of Factor VIII with VWF), replacement therapy is more complicated. For treat-

111

Table 4. Calculations of Doses of Factor Concentrate

Definitions

1. Target level: Level of factor desired for a given clinical situation (see Table 5).

2. Desired increment: Rise in factor level desired to increase factor level from the preinfusion level to the target level (measured in IU/dL, % or mg/dL)

3. Weight: Patient's weight in kilograms.

Estimation of dose is based on empiric observations in patients, with the desired increment multiplied by the patient's weight and divided by the empirically observed factor recovery. Dose is in IU (Factor VIII, Factor IX, antithrombin and protein C), in ristocetin cofactor units (von Willebrand factor) or milligrams (fibrinogen).

1. Factor VIII dose (IU) = (desired increment × weight)/2.0.

2. Factor IX (plasma-derived) dose = (desired increment × weight)/1.0.

3. Factor IX (recombinant) dose = (desired increment × weight)/0.76.

4. von Willebrand factor dose = (desired increment × weight)/1.5.

5. Antithrombin (plasma-derived) = (desired increment × weight)/1.4.

6. Protein C (plasma-derived) = (desired increment × weight)/1.4.

7. Fibrinogen (plasma-derived) = (desired increment × weight)/1.7.

Dose, frequency, and duration of therapy are dependent upon the severity of deficiency, patient's age, and clinical situation of the patient. See text and package inserts of the various factor preparations for further details.

ment of type 2N VWD, the recommended replacement concentrate must contain VWF. However, the dose calculations should be based on the product's labeled Factor VIII activity by using calculations appropriate for Factor VIII replacement (see sections on hemophilia, below). Finally, one must bear in mind that support of both the VWF and Factor VIII levels is required during the initial management of type 3 VWF, and dose calculations should take both hemostatic proteins into account.

Hemophilia A—Factor VIII Deficiency

Hemophilia A is an X-linked congenital bleeding disorder caused by Factor VIII deficiency. Gene deletions, gene rearrangements, and point mutations of the Factor VIII gene have been described.[15] The VWF levels are normal. The clinical severity of hemophilia is related to a patient's factor level. Severe hemophiliacs (defined as baseline Factor VIII levels below 1%) are at risk for spontaneous hemorrhage, whereas patients with factor levels above 5% are considered mild hemophiliacs, in whom significant trauma usually precedes bleeding episodes. Moderate hemophiliacs have Factor VIII levels of between 1% and 5% and may have excessive bleeding with minimal trauma or after surgery.

Unlike platelet-related bleeding, hemophilic bleeding manifests spontaneously or several hours after the causative trauma and occurs most frequently in deep structures such as joints and muscles. Bleeding may occur anywhere, however, including in the brain and the gastrointestinal tract.

Similar to VWD, mild hemophilia A can be treated with DDAVP, and the same principles of therapy apply.[15,29] Moderate or severe disease generally requires the infusion of Factor VIII concentrates. Recombinant Factor VIII concentrates are the products of choice followed by virus-inactivated plasma-derived Factor VIII (see Chapter 2: Plasma Derivatives). Cryoprecipitated AHF is used only in urgent situations when preferred concentrates are not immediately available. The duration of factor replacement therapy and target factor levels are dictated by the specific indications for treatment, severity of bleeding, and the patient's response to treatment (for examples of target values for various indications, see Table 5; more complete recommendations are available elsewhere[15,29]). Hemophilic joint bleeding is typically treated with Factor VIII replacement to a target level of

40% to 80%, with a follow-up infusion given the next day with the aim of achieving a follow-up increment of 40%. In preparation for surgery or when replacement therapy is required for management of a life-threatening event, the desired Factor VIII level is at least 100% of normal. After initial replacement, follow-up therapy is provided to maintain trough Factor VIII levels above 50%. The average half-life of infused Factor VIII is approximately 8 to 12 hours, so maintenance factor support may be accomplished by providing a dose of Factor VIII sufficient to provide a 50% increment every 12 hours. Although not licensed for continuous infusion, factor concentrate used in this fashion is becoming more common, especially in the postoperative setting. Continuous infusion therapy allows more stable factor levels and simplifies monitoring while also using less concentrate.[15] Infusion is typically initiated at approximately 4 IU/kg/hour, and the dose is then titrated based on laboratory monitoring.[30]

Factor products are available as lyophilized concentrate. The quantity of Factor VIII coagulant activity is stated on the vial label in terms of international units (IU). One IU is the amount of Factor VIII coagulant activity present in 1 mL of normal plasma.

Table 5. Initial Target Factor Levels for Various Clinical Situations (unit/dL) and Half-Life of Infused Material

Clinical Situation	Factor VIII	Factor IX	VWF
Life-threatening bleeding or surgery	80-100	60-80	80-100
Hemophilic joint bleeding	80	60	NA
Minor bleeding event	40	30	30
Half-life (hours)	8-12	20-24	8-12

VWF = von Willebrand factor; NA = not available. Target level and frequency of follow-up doses should be decided according to the clinical situation, factor half-life, and other clinical variables. For further details, refer to references 15, 25, 26, and 29.

The method of calculation for dosing that is generally used by hematologists involves the empiric observation that each unit of Factor VIII infused per kilogram of body weight yields a 2% rise in the plasma Factor VIII level (ie, 0.02 IU/mL or 2 IU/dL; see Table 4). In hospitalized patients who require repeated infusions, the Factor VIII levels should be monitored to ensure adequate replacement. Approximately 10% to 15% of patients with severe hemophilia A develop neutralizing immunoglobulin G (IgG) antibodies after repeated Factor VIII infusions.[31] These patients with inhibitors require therapeutic products that have Factor VIII-bypassing activity (see Management of Inhibitors to Factor VIII or Factor IX, below). Treatment of hemophilic bleeding is best managed in conjunction with an experienced consultant who is familiar with the care of this complicated condition.

Hemophilia B—Factor IX Deficiency

The inheritance and clinical manifestations of Factor IX deficiency are identical to those of Factor VIII deficiency. Although the principles of replacement therapy are similar for these disorders, several specific differences must be pointed out. DDAVP and Cryoprecipitated AHF are *not* effective in the treatment of patients with Factor IX deficiency; replacement therapy for patients with hemophilia B requires the infusion of products that contain Factor IX. Although concentrates are available from either plasma-derived or recombinant sources, most hemophilia treatment centers in the United States rely on recombinant material (BeneFix, Wyeth, Philadelphia, PA). Dosing schedules for Factor IX vary from those for Factor VIII, because of the differences in the two factors' hemostatic effectiveness, volume of distribution, and half-life (see Tables 4 and 5). In the initial treatment of hemophilic joint hemorrhage, the target Factor IX level is 30% to 60%, and the follow-up dose administered the next day is targeted to achieve an increment of 30%. In preparation for surgery or when replacement therapy is required for the management of a life-threatening event, the desired Factor IX level is at least 80% of normal. After initial replacement, follow-up therapy is provided to maintain trough Factor IX levels above 40%. The empirical method of calculation for dosing of plasma-derived Factor IX concentrate is based on the observation that the infusion of 1 unit of human plasma-derived Factor IX per kilogram of body weight yields a 1% increment of plasma Factor IX level (ie, 0.01 IU/mL or 1 IU/dL). Recombinant Factor IX has a somewhat lower recovery than does plasma-derived Factor IX. For that reason, most physicians increase the dose by 1.3 to 1.5 times when the recombinant material is used. The average half-life of infused Factor IX is approximately 18 to 24 hours, and thus maintenance factor support may be administered daily or via continuous infusion.[15,29] Factor levels should be monitored in patients who require repeated infusions.

Approximately 1% to 4% of hemophilia B patients develop inhibitors (antibodies) to Factor IX. These antibodies generally develop early in their clinical history and may be associated with anaphylactic reactions.[31] A bleeding hemophilia B patient with an inhibitor may respond to recombinant Factor VIIa (see Management of Inhibitors to Factor VIII or Factor IX, below).

Management of Inhibitors to Factor VIII or Factor IX

Development of inhibitory antibodies to a coagulation factor is a serious consequence of factor replacement therapy. Patients with low titers of inhibitors (less than 5 Bethesda units) may achieve satisfactory responses to increased doses of factor, but this approach is generally fruitless in patients with higher titer inhibitors. Immune tolerance therapy, aimed at eradication of the inhibitor antibody through daily infusions of high doses of Factor VIII or IX, has been successful in producing tolerance in up to 70% of hemophilia A patients but in only 30% of hemophilia B patients.[29,31]

Factor products that possess "bypassing activity," such as activated prothrombin complex concentrates (aPCCs) or recombinant Factor VIIa,[31] are the mainstay of therapy for patients with inhibitors. The precise mechanism of action of an aPCC (such as FEIBA-NF, Baxter, Westlake Village CA) is unclear, but evidence points to the activation of Factor X and prothrombin, which bypasses the role of Factor VIII in the coagulation mechanism. The initial dose of 50 to 100 units/kg can be repeated in 6 to 12 hours, but thrombotic complications have been reported with repeated use of aPCCs. Concurrent use of antifibrinolytics should therefore be avoided with these agents. The FDA-approved use of recombinant Factor VIIa (rFVIIa, NovoSeven, NovoNordisk, Bagsvaerd, Denmark) as a bypassing agent for the treatment of inhibitor patients.[31] The primary mechanisms of action appear to involve TF-dependent activation of Factor X and TF-independent activation of Factors IX and X on the surface of activated platelets. The licensed recommended dose is 90 µg/kg, but more recent investigations have explored the use of doses as high as 200 to 300 µg/kg. In the treatment of inhibitor patients, rFVIIa has had few adverse side effects and a low risk of thrombosis.[32] Drawbacks of using bypassing agents include expense, absence of a laboratory monitor for treatment efficacy, and a short plasma half-life (estimated at 2.7 hours for rFVIIa). No therapy is universally successful in the management of hemophilia patients with inhibitors, and consultation with a physician experienced in the care of these challenging patients is prudent.

In rare instances, spontaneous Factor VIII inhibitors occur as an autoimmune process in previously normal individuals. These autoantibodies are mainly seen in the postpartum setting or in elderly patients with associated autoimmune or malignant disease. Patients usually present with severe bleeding and are managed in a fashion similar to that for hemophilia patients with inhibitors, but in addition, immunotherapy aimed at suppression of autoantibody is also required. Inhibitors to other coagulation factors occur very rarely.

Factor XI Deficiency

In Factor XI deficiency, the bleeding tendency varies widely among individuals and is poorly correlated with factor level. Mucosal bleeding and menorrhagia are the most frequent presenting symptoms. Diagnosis may be complicated by the fact that many aPTT assays are insensitive to mild Factor XI deficiency; if this disease is suspected, specific measurement of Factor XI is suggested. Although extensive hemorrhage can occur after trauma or surgery, some patients have tolerated surgery without excessive bleeding despite an almost undetectable Factor XI level; an individual patient's history of clinical bleeding in comparison to hemostatic challenge should be reviewed as one decides on the need for factor replacement before a surgical procedure. Factor XI concentrate is not available in the United States and treatment with plasma to achieve a Factor XI level 30% to 45% of normal is sufficient for hemostasis in most situations. Factor XI has a half-life of 52 ± 22 hours. DDAVP and antifibrinolytic agents may be considered for minor mucosal bleeding.[33]

Other Factor Deficiencies

Deficiencies of vitamin-K-dependent Factors II, VII, or X and deficiency of the non-vitamin-K-dependent Factors V and XIII are rare causes of congenital bleeding diathesis. With the notable exceptions of Factor XI (discussed above) and Factor VII, the severity of bleeding manifestations is generally correlated with a patient's measured factor level.

Recombinant Factor VIIa is the replacement product of choice for treatment of congenital Factor VII deficiency.[34] Although the half-life of rFVIIa is about 3 hours (similar to nonactivated Factor VII), doses of 15 to 30 μg/kg administered at intervals of 4 to 6 hours have been successful. Whole-blood-derived plasma is commonly used for replacement therapy in patients with deficiency of either Factor II (prothrombin) or Factor X; however, PCC could be considered as a virus-attenuated alternative. PCCs contain variable amounts of all of the vitamin-K-dependent factors, but there is a paradoxical risk for thrombosis when PCCs are used. For both Factors II and X, a level of approximately 30 U/dL is generally considered sufficient for surgery. It is estimated that infusion of 1 U/kg would increase the prothrombin level by 1 U/dL, while recovery of Factor X is slightly greater at

1.5 U/dL. Both Factor II and Factor X have a long postinfusion half-life (72-96 hours and 40-60 hours, respectively).

For patients with congenital deficiency of the non-vitamin-K-dependent Factor V, preoperative levels of 25% to 30% are recommended. Although Factor V is called "labile factor," it is only minimally decreased in Plasma Frozen Within 24 Hours After Phlebotomy or Thawed Plasma.[35,36] Patients with congenital Factor XII deficiency have no bleeding symptoms and do not require replacement therapy.

Severe Factor XIII deficiency is a severe bleeding disorder that often presents with umbilical stump bleeding, but is also associated with a high risk of spontaneous intracranial hemorrrhage. PT, PTT, and fibrinogen assays are normal, and specific tests of Factor XIII function (either clot solubility or quantitative Factor XIII assay) will confirm a diagnosis. Replacement is achieved with pasteurized concentrate (Corifact, CSL Behring, King of Prussia, PA), and although Cryoprecipitated AHF also contains Factor XIII,[28] it is no longer the preferred replacement.[37] Factor XIII has a long half-life (5-11 days). Levels should be maintained above 5% to prevent spontaneous intracranial hemorrhage, but higher levels (at least 10-25%) are suggested for surgery. Inherited disorders of fibrinogen may be quantitative or qualitative. In patients with congenital defects, fibrinogen replacement therapy may be indicated to treat or prevent surgical bleeding, improve wound healing, or prevent recurrent pregnancy loss. The FDA has licensed a heat-treated fibrinogen concentrate (RiaSTAP) for patients with congenital fibrinogen deficiency; however, cryoprecipitate remains the FDA-licensed product for use in other settings.[28] Fibrinogen has a long half-life (55-120 hours) and suggested minimum target levels are 50 mg/dL to prevent recurrent pregnancy loss, and over 100 mg/dL in surgical settings.[38]

Alpha$_2$-Plasmin Inhibitor

Deficiency of alpha$_2$-plasmin inhibitor, the primary circulating plasmin inhibitor, is associated with a severe hemorrhagic disorder. Diagnosis requires a specific assay for this inhibitor. Therapy consists of replacement by plasma transfusion and/or oral antifibrinolytic agents such as epsilon aminocaproic acid (EACA).[39]

Acquired Bleeding Disorders

Vitamin K Deficiency and Vitamin K Antagonists

Vitamin K is a fat-soluble vitamin that is necessary for synthesis in the liver of coagulation Factors II, VII, IX, and X, protein C, and protein S. Nutritional deficiency states can occur in patients in the intensive care unit, those who have chronic disease and are receiving antibiotics, and those with general fat-malabsorption states, such as celiac disease, pancreatic insufficiency, or obstructive jaundice. The dose and route of vitamin K administration depend on the clinical situation. Oral administration is preferred over subcutaneous administration because of the delayed and unpredictable response to subcutaneously administered vitamin K.[40] Intravenous infusion of vitamin K has been associated, rarely, with anaphylaxis, but a slow infusion rate reduces the risk for patients in whom the oral route is unavailable. The full effect of vitamin K is achieved only after 12 to 24 hours; thus, urgent correction of deficiencies of the vitamin-K-dependent factors requires factor infusion in addition to vitamin K replacement (see below).

Oral anticoagulants, such as warfarin, are the mainstay of outpatient anticoagulation therapy, interfering with the vitamin-K-dependent synthesis of coagulation Factors II, VII, IX, and X. Despite their effectiveness, vitamin K antagonists are plagued with problems, including a narrow therapeutic window, considerable dose-response variability between patients, interactions with both drugs and dietary factors, and difficulty in maintaining a therapeutic degree of anticoagulation [as monitored by the international normalized ratio (INR)]. In rare cases, warfarin-induced skin necrosis can develop about 1 to 4 days after initiation of therapy, and it is related to the drug's early inhibition of production of a coagulation regulatory factor (protein C). Patients with congenital deficiency of protein C or its cofactor (protein S) are at increased risk for the development of this complication of warfarin therapy and may warrant coverage with heparin-based therapy until the full warfarin effect is achieved. Warfarin overdose is treated by withdrawal of the drug and/or the administration of vitamin K.[40] In the absence of bleeding, 0.5 to 2 mg of oral vitamin K may be sufficient, but 5 to 10 mg is recommended when the INR is more than 9. For serious bleeding in which either vitamin K deficiency or warfarin effect is a confounding issue, factor replacement therapy may be required in addition to vitamin K administration. This can be accomplished by large-volume (up to 2 liters) transfusion of plasma, but volume overload and time delays are common. Recently, off-label use of PCC in the urgent reversal of vitamin K antagonists has become more common, as PCC is clearly a more efficient option. The three-factor PCC commonly available in the United States lacks sufficient Factor VII to correct a prolonged INR, and supplementation with either plasma or rFVIIa has been advocated.[41] PCC is generally labeled by its Factor IX content, and dosing algorithms of PCC have been proposed based on the patient's weight and INR[40,41]; however, some centers have simplified ordering to weight-based prescription. Case reports suggest that rFVIIa can be used alone (off-label) as an alternative to PCC; this results in replacement of only one of the deficient coagulation factors. Additional drawbacks include the short half-life and potential for thrombotic complications associated with rFVIIa.[40,42]

Liver Disease

Patients with liver disease have multiple coagulation derangements, including coagulation factor deficiencies, impaired vitamin K utilization, and activated fibrinolysis. Thrombocytopenia may add to the bleeding diathesis, and it is usually the result of multiple factors that include hypersplenism, increased platelet consumption, and diminished hepatic thrombopoietin production. These hemostatic abnormalities do not by themselves lead to spontaneous bleeding, but may increase the risk and severity of bleeding related to operative procedures or complications of portal hypertension. Patients with liver disease and mild coagulopathy are sensitive to dilutional coagulopathy. Thus, treatment with plasma (10-20 mL/kg) is reasonable in liver disease patients with coagulopathy when bleeding is present, because further dilution of coagulation factors is expected with the infusion of replacement red cells or plasma-free solutions. Liver biopsy, paracentesis, and thoracentesis are common diagnostic procedures in patients with liver disease, but there is a paucity of data to suggest that mild abnormalities of INR predict periprocedural bleeding. Furthermore, correction of the INR is often not accomplished with the volume of plasma product infused.[12,13] Data are scarce regarding the threshold for platelet transfusion before liver biopsy, but some institutions use a platelet count of 50,000/μL.[12] Alternative approaches to liver biopsy such as transvenous approach, or "plugging" should be considered to decrease the risk of bleeding with liver biopsy. It is important to note that patients with hepatic failure may require larger volumes of plasma than do other patients to achieve PT improvement. Correction of coagulation tests after plasma transfusion may not be complete in patients with liver disease, because of the presence of fibrin fragments, dysfibrinogenemia, and rapid movement of factors into the extravascular space. The value of rFVIIa for decreasing transfusion requirement in bleeding patients with cirrhosis has been explored in multiple settings, but well-conducted clinical trials have generally shown little advantage to the use of this approach.[12,42]

Disseminated Intravascular Coagulation

A multitude of disorders, including infections, malignancy, and inflammatory conditions lead to activation of the coagulation mechanism. If the activation overwhelms compensatory mechanisms, the clinical syndrome of DIC becomes manifest. Increased degradation of coagulation proteins and protease inhibitors, and widespread microvascular thrombosis, leads to depletion of coagulation proteins and platelets.[43] The diagnosis of DIC requires integration of both clinical and laboratory data. The chief clinical manifestation in the acute form of DIC is organ dysfunction, but bleeding or thrombotic events may also require clinical attention. Routinely employed laboratory tests are neither sensitive nor specific for diagnosis of DIC, and thus a panel of studies is usually needed to make the diagnosis. Serial measurement of PT, aPTT, platelet count, and fibrinogen level to identify progressive reduction in coagulation components is helpful to establish the diagnosis and guide therapy in this dynamically changing condition. Thrombocytopenia is present in 80% to 90% of cases and D-dimer is elevated in 99%. Vigorous treatment of the underlying disease, correction of acidosis, and aggressive support of tissue perfusion are the cornerstones of therapy. In the bleeding patient (or one requiring an invasive procedure), the transfusion of platelets, plasma, and/or Cryoprecipitated AHF should be guided by clinical features and laboratory values. Specific thresholds for transfusion are not established, but maintaining a platelet count over 50,000/μL and a fibrinogen level over 100 mg/dL has been suggested.[44] If thrombosis and tissue ischemia are prominent, heparin may be used to inhibit thrombin generation. Antithrombin concentrate has not been demonstrated to improve any clinically relevant endpoint; however, infusion of recombinant activated protein C (Xigris, Eli Lilly, Indianapolis, IN) decreased mortality in patients with severe sepsis, and post-hoc analysis revealed that patients with DIC had the highest benefit.[43] Potent antifibrinolytic or prohemostatic agents (such as EACA or rFVIIa) are generally not recommended in patients with DIC, as they theoretically could increase the thrombotic risk.

Dilutional Coagulopathy and Refractory Surgical Bleeding

In patients with extensive trauma or surgery, lost blood is usually initially replaced with large volumes of crystalloid solution in order to maintain circulating blood volume. This may result in the substantial dilution of blood platelets and plasma coagulation factors. The coupling of hemodilution with hypoperfusion-related acidosis and hypothermia worsens the coagulation defect in trauma and massively transfused patients. This acquired coagulation disturbance is exacerbated by the transfusion of Red Blood Cell (RBC) units because they lack functional platelets and significant amounts of coagulation factors. The correlation between the number of RBC units infused and the dilution of coagulation factors and platelets is imprecise. Furthermore, many labs are unable to generate conventional monitoring data (PT, PTT, fibrinogen, and platelet count) quickly enough to meet the needs of physicians caring for these unstable and rapidly bleeding patients. Military and civilian hospital data suggest that in the massively transfused trauma patient, empiric hemostatic product support results in decreased mortality.[45] Level I trauma centers are required to maintain a "massive transfusion protocol" whereby transfusion of platelets and plasma is prescribed in a fixed ratio to RBC transfusion.[16] The optimal balance between RBCs, platelets, and plasma components remains to be established, and prospective studies to confirm current observational data are pending. Anecdotal reports suggest the utility of rFVIIa in the trauma setting, however, a controlled trial did not demonstrate a survival advantage.[42] Despite the growing enthusiasm for massive transfusion protocols, the role of ongoing clinical assessment and laboratory monitoring to inform transfusion decisions should not be abandoned. Novel methods to improve laboratory turnaround times and communication of data are emerging, and nonconventional point-of-care testing (such as thromboelastography) are finding their way into clinical practice guidelines.[16,20] Extrapolation from elective surgical settings suggests that reasonable transfusion thresholds in an actively bleeding patient may be a platelet count of 50,000/µL, fibrinogen level of 100 mg/dL, and PT-INR of 1.6 or greater.[46]

Anticoagulant Drugs

Vitamin K antagonists (such as warfarin) have been the mainstay of outpatient anticoagulation and were discussed earlier in this chapter.

Heparin-based drugs [either conventional unfractionated heparin (UFH) or low-molecular-weight heparin (LMWH) derivatives] are among the most frequently prescribed medications to treat or prevent thromboembolism. Heparin markedly enhances the ability of antithrombin to neutralize serine proteases. Even slight contamination of the diagnostic sample with UFH (eg, the flush volume in a subclavian catheter) can prolong the TT and the aPTT, which can lead to confusion in diagnosis. The risk of bleeding in patients taking heparin drugs is modified by many factors, including comorbid conditions (such as recent surgery, trauma, or renal failure), the patient's age and gender, and the use of concomitant antiplatelet drugs.[47] Plasma is not effective in reversing UFH effect, and acute heparin reversal is accomplished with protamine sulfate.[40] At the completion of cardiac bypass surgery, algorithms or point-of-care testing can be used to estimate the quantity of circulating heparin in order to select an appropriate protamine dose; 1 mg of protamine sulfate neutralizes 80 to 100 units of UFH. Protamine has a shorter half-life than UFH, and "rebound" heparin effect or initial underestimations of the protamine dose should be considered in a patient with unexplained bleeding after protamine therapy.[27] LMWH is derived by enzymatic or chemical depolymerization of UFH. FDA-approved indications and dose schedules differ between the various approved LMWH preparations, but, as a class, they share most attributes. LMWH drugs have less anti-Factor IIa activity (and thus less effect on the aPTT) than does UFH, but they retain the ability to accelerate antithrombin effect against Factor Xa, and thus they remain potent anticoagulant drugs. Compared to UFH, LMWH produces a more predictable anticoagulant response, has a longer plasma half-life (3 to 12 hours), and fewer interactions with osteoclasts and platelets. These qualities translate into weight-based dosing on a once- to twice-daily time frame, no need to monitor levels in most patient settings, and a reduced risk for HIT. The aPTT is not an appropriate monitor of LMWH effect, and specific drug levels (via anti-Factor Xa assay) are required if monitoring is desired. LMWH is cleared mainly through a renal mechanism, and dose adjustment is required in patients with significant renal impairment. If excessive bleeding occurs, protamine may be helpful but it is not a completely effective antidote.

Fondaparinux (Arixtra, GlaxoSmithKline, Research Triangle Park, NC) is a synthetic pentasaccharide that strongly binds antithrombin and acts as a selective inhibitor to Factor Xa. It is administered parenterally, has a half-life of 17 to 21 hours, and is cleared primarily through renal secretion. Clinical licensing has been for thromboprophylaxis in the orthopedic setting and for initial treatment of venous thrombotic disease; dose schedules are weight-based and do not rely on drug level monitoring. Fondaparinux is not neutralized by protamine and is not easily removed via dialysis. Case reports suggest that off-label use of rFVIIa has been helpful in patients who develop severe bleeding complications while on Fondaparinux.[40]

Direct-acting coagulation factor inhibitors are an emerging class of medications. Three parenterally administered direct thrombin inhibitors (DTIs) have been available for several years.[48] Argatroban (Texas Biotechnology, Houston, TX) is a competitive inhibitor of thrombin that acts via noncovalent interaction with thrombin. It is administered by continuous infusion and has a plasma half-life of approximately 45 minutes, but clearance is very prolonged in patients with hepatic dysfunction (even if this is caused by passive congestion after cardiac surgery). Lepirudin (Refludan, Berlex Laboratories, Montville, NJ) and bivalirudin (Angiomax, The Medicines Co., Parsippany, NJ) are both recombinant peptide drugs based upon the amino acid sequence of hirudin, the anticoagulant protein present in the salivary secretions of the medicinal leech. Lepirudin has a half-life of approximately 80 minutes, is cleared through a renal route, and is indicated for the management of HIT. Bivalirudin has a few advantages over lepirudin, in that its binding to thrombin is reversible and it has a shorter plasma half-life (approximately 25 minutes). Bivalirudin is partially cleared by the kidney, and the remaining clearance occurs via proteolysis. It is indicated for treatment during acute coronary angioplasty and in unstable angina. Bleeding complications that arise during the use of DTI drugs must be handled by drug discontinuation. The therapeutic efficacy of rFVIIa in this setting has been disappointing.[40]

Development of oral direct-acting coagulation inhibitors ("Xabans") is now coming to fruition. Their rapid onset of action, predictable pharmacokinetic profile, broader therapeutic window, and relative lack of interactions with other medications make them an attractive alternative to vitamin-K antagonists. Clinical studies in thromboprophylaxis, prevention of systemic thromboembolism in the setting of atrial fibrillation, and prevention of recurrent venous thromboembolic (VTE) disease, have generally shown superiority or at least noninferiority compared with vitamin-K antagonists or LMWH. Clinical laboratory monitoring of anticoagulant effect was not performed in these trials and is not a recommended component of patient care algorithms that use these agents. The major disadvantages of these agents includes the absence of a drug antidote and absence of established guidelines related to management of acute bleeding complications. Dabigatran (Pradaxa, Boeringer Ingelheim, Ridgefield, CT) is an example of an oral DTI. Its half-life is 14 to 17 hours in patients with normal renal function. Routine coagulation tests are of limited value in assessing anticoagulant effect; however, the PTT is usually prolonged on therapy, and the thrombin clot time is exquisitely sensitive in demonstrating that drug is present. Rivaroxaban (Xarleto, Bayer Inc, Pittsburgh, PA) is an example of an oral direct Factor Xa inhibitor. It has a half-life of 5 to 9 hours in younger patients, but 11 to 13 hours in individuals over 75 years of age. Drug elimination is primarily renal, but 1/3 is excreted in feces. Both PT and PTT are prolonged on therapy, and the drug level may be estimated by either PT or anti-

Xa assay using a standard curve calibrated with dilutions of the medication. Dabigatran and rivaroxaban should be discontinued at least 24 hours before elective surgery to allow the drug to clear, but this interval should be adjusted based upon the degree of renal function and surgical bleeding risk.[49,50] There are currently very limited options for patients receiving these anticoagulants who present with bleeding complications. These include local hemostatic maneuvers (such as mechanical compression and surgical hemostasis), and supportive care until the drug is cleared. Hemodialysis will accelerate clearance of dabigatran. There is no clinical evidence that plasma products will reverse the anticoagulant effect of direct coagulation factor inhibitors, but preclinical studies suggest a potential role for rFVIIa, PCC, or activated PCC.[49,50]

Application of antiplatelet drug therapy has expanded greatly, owing to a greater appreciation of the role of platelets in arterial thrombotic disease and a growing understanding of platelet physiology.[8,51] Aspirin has multiple favorable properties. For most patients, daily low-dose aspirin is sufficient to inhibit the action of platelet cyclooxygenase, providing platelet inhibition by preventing the generation of thromboxane A_2. Although aspirin does not completely inhibit platelet function, it has the advantages of the oral route, low expense, and the presence of vast clinical experience. Disadvantages include an estimated incidence of major gastrointestinal hemorrhage of one to two per 1000 patient-years and the recent recognition of inter-individual variation in effectiveness (so-called "aspirin resistance"). Metabolic derivatives of thienopyridine drugs such as clopidogrel (Plavix, Bristol-Myers Squibb/Sanofi Pharmaceuticals, New York, NY) and prasugrel (Effient, Eli Lilly, Indianapolis, IN) selectively inhibit ADP-induced activation of platelets via irreversible alteration of the platelet P_2Y_{12} receptor. Similar to aspirin, thienopyridines are administered by repeated oral dosing, which is sometimes initiated with a larger loading dose. Clopidogrel's effect lasts approximately 7 days. Inhibitors of platelet activation are only partially effective, and a class of more potent platelet inhibitory drugs relies on interrupting the final common pathway of platelet aggregation via inhibition of the platelet fibrinogen receptor (GPIIb-IIIa). Abciximab (ReoPro, Eli Lilly, Indianapolis, IN) is a recombinant chimeric antibody fragment with a functional effect that lasts approximately 48 hours after infusion. Peptide analogs of the sequence of fibrinogen that binds GPIIb-IIIa include epifibatide (Integrilin, Merck Pharmaceutical, Whitehorse Station, NJ) and tirofiban (Aggrestat, Merck Pharmaceutical, Whitehorse Station, NJ). Epifibatide (a cyclic heptapeptide) and tirofiban (a peptidomimetic drug) have a short plasma half-life, and drug infusions are used if continued prolonged platelet inhibition is required. Bleeding complications that occur during use of the glycoprotein receptor-inhibiting drugs are managed with discontinuation of the medication. Platelet transfusion may be required for reversal of medication effect (especially with abciximab, which has a long-lasting effect) and for treatment of the rare patient who develops severe thrombocytopenia as a complication of the use of these potent drugs.[51]

Prohemostatic Drugs

DDAVP is a synthetic analog of vasopressin, which is a selective V2 receptor agonist. Its mechanism of action as a prohemostatic agent is incompletely understood, but mainly attributed to stimulation of the endothelial cells, with subsequent endothelial cell release of granular contents (VWF, Factor VIII, and tissue plasminogen activator) and activation of nitric oxide synthetase. DDAVP has been used primarily in the treatment of mild inherited or acquired platelet function defects, hemophilia A, and VWD. It is usually administered intravenously at a dose of 0.3 μg/kg over 20 minutes, or as a concentrated nasal spray designed for outpatient use (Stimate, CSL Behring, King of Prussia, PA). DDAVP has been studied as a tool for blood conservation in patients without underlying hemostatic defects undergoing elective cardiac or orthopedic surgery. Review of these studies fails to support the routine use of DDAVP in this setting. but it may be helpful in the subset of patients taking aspirin.[4,27]

The antifibrinolytic drugs that are available take the form of either synthetic lysine analogs, or protein-based inhibitors. EACA (Amicar, Xanodyne Pharmaceuticals, Newport, KY) and tranexamic acid (Lysteda, Ferring Pharmaceuticals, Saint-Prex, Switzerland) are synthetic lysine analogs. Through occupancy of lysine binding sites of both plasminogen and the plasminogen activators, these agents delay clot resorption. Oral secretions are rich in plasminogen activators. Antifibrinolytic agents are useful as an adjunctive therapy in patients with bleeding disorders who require dental procedures and topical administration may provide therapeutic effect while avoiding systemic toxicities. The anhepatic phase of liver transplantation is another setting in which intense fibrinolysis may result in bleeding complications; studies support a positive effect of antifibrinolytic agents in that setting. Antifibrinolytic agents have been shown to decrease blood loss in the cardiac surgery setting, and meta-analysis of studies confirmed both a decreased rate of surgical re-exploration and decreased mortality in cardiac surgery patients.[4] Similarly, these medications might be considered for control of bleeding in patients requiring support with extracorporeal membrane oxygenation (ECMO). Other recommendations related to ECMO-related bleeding include maintaining platelet count greater than 80,000/μL, fibrinogen level more than 250 mg/dL, and maintaining adequate antithrombin and hemoglobin levels.[4] Antifibrinolytic agents have also been used in the management of thrombocytopenic bleeding (eg, patients with immune thrombocytopenia and myelosuppressed patients refractory to platelet transfusion), but the results have been inconsistent in thrombocytopenic patients.[27] Tranexamic acid is 6 to 10 times more potent on a molar basis, but is currently less available in the United States. Both drugs are water soluble, cleared through a renal mechanism, and have a relatively short half-life. The principal adverse effect of EACA is gastrointestinal intolerance, commonly presenting as nausea, cramps, or diarrhea. Hypotension may occur with rapid intravenous administration, and myopathy is a rare complication of prolonged use. Thrombosis has generally not been a complication of EACA use in the hemophilic or perioperative setting, but is a significant risk in the setting of DIC.[27]

Aprotinin is a protein obtained from bovine lung that inhibits fibrinolysis through inhibition of plasmin activity. Although shown to decrease perioperative bleeding and the transfusion requirement of patients undergoing cardiac surgery, three independent cohort studies have recently suggested increased complications and mortality in cardiac surgery patients who received this agent. These safety concerns have resulted in the manufacturer of this agent restricting marketing at the current time.[4]

Conjugated estrogens have been used to augment hemostasis in a wide variety of settings including uremia and patients with chronic bleeding associated with hereditary hemorrhagic telangiectasia or angiodysplasia. Oral contraceptive is a first-line therapy for controlling menorrhagia in women with VWD, and hormonal manipulation is often used to prevent this complication in reproductive-age women undergoing myeloablative chemotherapy.[27]

Topical hemostatic agents are useful to control localized bleeding. A large array of materials are available. Topical compressive agents include oxidized regenerated cellulose and microfibrillar collagen. Anastomotic sealants contain thrombin, which may be compounded with fibrinogen and antifibrinolytics in the form of fibrin sealant.

Thrombophilia

Thrombophilia is a term used by clinicians to describe venous or arterial thromboembolism that develops spontaneously, at an early age, or at an unusual site, and involves recurrent thrombotic events. It is multifactorial, and most thrombophilia patients have several acquired and genetic risk factors.[18] The list of currently recognized inherited thrombophilic defects includes deficiency of coagulation control proteins (ie, antithrombin, protein C, and protein S), subtle defects of coagulation control (eg, Factor V Leiden), and increased levels of coagulation factors (probably the mechanism underlying the Prothrombin G20210A). Elevation of Factor VIII and homocysteine levels may involve both inherited and acquired factors. The list of acquired prothrombotic states is long, but it can be broken down into circumstantial factors (eg, advanced age, immobility, pregnancy, and hormone replacement therapy) and disease-related factors (eg, surgery, malignancy, presence of an intravascular device, antiphospholipid syndrome, and HIT). The most common manifestation is VTE disease, which presents as either deep vein thrombosis or pulmonary embolism. Thrombophilic defects also contribute to the risk of VTE recurrence, and their presence is taken into account in planning the duration of long-term anticoagulation in patients who have experienced thrombosis.[18] Patients with a history of symptomatic thrombophilia should be considered for thromboprophylaxis during periods of increased risk, such as surgery or pregnancy.[52-54]

Genetic and serologic evaluations of thrombophilia are not affected by anticoagulation, but tests of plasma coagulation factors are best delayed until the effects of acute thrombosis have passed and anticoagulation is completed. Antithrombin, protein C, and protein S levels may transiently decrease and fibrinogen and Factor VIII may increase in response to an acute thrombotic episode. Heparin therapy may depress antithrombin levels, and complicates the interpretation of some assays for lupus anticoagulant. Warfarin therapy may also complicate interpretation of assays for lupus anticoagulant and it suppresses protein C and protein S levels; protein S levels may not return to baseline for up to 4 to 6 weeks after discontinuing warfarin.[55]

Transfusion support of patients with thrombophilia is rarely required. However, replacement therapy might be considered in situations where anticoagulant drug therapy presents an unacceptable bleeding risk or is unsuccessful (see below).

Deficiency of Coagulation Control Proteins

Antithrombin is the most important protease inhibitor of activated coagulation factors and is central to the in-vivo effect of heparin-based anticoagulants. Both human-plasma-derived, virus-inactivated antithrombin concentrate (Thrombate III, Talecris Biotherapeutics, Research Triangle Park, NC) and recombinant antithrombin (Atryn, GTC Biotherapeutics, Farmington, MA) are available; however, the recombinant material has a much shorter half-life, such that continuous infusion is recommended when that preparation is chosen. Replacement therapy is approved for treatment of patients with hereditary antithrombin deficiency in connection with surgery or parturition, when the risk of anticoagulant therapy may be considered unacceptable. Antithrombin replacement has also been used in settings where achievement of anticoagulation with heparin has proven difficult, but published evidence is limited.[4,55]

Heterozygous deficiencies of protein C and protein S, two vitamin-K-dependent anticoagulant proteins, are associated with recurrent thromboembolic disease. Homozygotes present with purpura fulminans as infants. Symptomatic patients are generally managed with anticoagulation. Initiation of warfarin anticoagulation is associated with an increased risk for development of warfarin-induced skin necrosis, and concomitant heparin therapy is suggested during this interval. Replacement therapy may be useful in some situations. Human-plasma-derived protein C concentrate (Ceprotin, Baxter Healthcare, Westlake Village, CA) is available for treatment and prophylaxis of patients with severe protein C deficiency presenting with purpura fulminans or venous thrombosis.[56] Isolated case reports suggest that protein C concentrate or activated protein C concentrate (Xigris, Eli Lilly, Indianapolis, IN) may also improve the outcome of patients with purpura fulminans associated with meningococcal sepsis.

Antiphospholipid Syndrome

Antiphospholipid syndrome is a clinical entity in which patients present with symptoms of thrombosis (either arterial or venous), recurrent pregnancy loss, or thrombocytopenia; there also exists laboratory evidence of autoantibodies that appear targeted to a variety of phospholipid-binding proteins.[57] Although anticardiolipin is a clinically useful screening serologic assay, beta-2 glycoprotein I appears to be the relevant epitope in the assay. Prothrombin and annexin V are other potentially important antibody targets. Antiphospholipid antibodies also may interfere with the assembly of coagulation factors on phospholipid surfaces in vitro, manifesting as a coagulation inhibitor known as a "lupus anticoagulant." The choice of the name lupus anticoagulant is unfortunate, because many of the patients with this entity do not have systemic lupus erythematosus and these antibodies are clinically associated with thrombosis. Laboratory diagnostic criteria for a lupus anticoagulant require 1) detection of a prolonged phospholipid-dependent coagulation time (usually both the aPTT and the dilute Russell viper venom time are tested); 2) incomplete correction of the prolonged clotting test by using a 1:1 mixture of patient plasma with normal plasma (demonstrating the presence of a coagulation inhibitor); and 3) correction of the prolonged clotting time upon addition of excess phospholipid (demonstrating phospholipid dependence). If the patient experiences clinical bleeding, then the absence of a specific factor deficiency or inhibitor should also be demonstrated. This last criterion is crucial because lupus anticoagulants are generally not associated with clinical bleeding unless prothrombin (Factor II) levels are also diminished (a diagnosis meriting evaluation if the PT is prolonged), and because Factor VIII inhibitors may confound interpretation of aPTT-based assays used to diagnose lupus anticoagulant.

Transfusion therapy for patients with antiphospholipid syndrome is rarely required. Situations where this might arise include surgical interventions or bleeding in patients with associated thrombocytopenia, or in patients with catastrophic antiphospholipid syndrome—a multi-organ failure syndrome associated with a high mortality rate in which treatment strategies include a combination of immune suppression, antithrombotic therapy, and therapeutic plasma exchange (TPE) [American Society for Apheresis (ASFA) indication Category III].[58] Occasionally, bleeding is attributable to autoimmune prothrombin deficiency complicating antiphospholipid syndrome; in this setting immune suppression is the principal intervention, but case reports suggest rFVIIa or plasma exchange may provide value in urgent settings.[59]

Heparin-Induced Thrombocytopenia

HIT is a drug-associated immune thrombocytopenic disorder characterized by paradoxical thrombosis. The decline in platelet count generally occurs between days 4 and 14 of heparin-based therapy, decreasing to below 50% of the pretreatment level. Thrombotic risk is very high in this condition, and asymptomatic thrombosis should be considered in patients with HIT. If HIT is suspected, heparin should be promptly discontinued, diagnostic evaluation should be initiated (such as platelet factor 4 enzyme immunoassay), and an alternative immediate-acting anticoagulant (eg, DTIs such as lepirudin or argatroban) should be substituted to provide anticoagulation.[22,60] Platelet transfusion is generally avoided in this condition, as bleeding complications are rare, and platelet transfusion may exacerbate the thrombotic tendency.

Thrombotic Thrombocytopenia Purpura

TTP is a clinical syndrome characterized by widespread microvascular thrombosis resulting in consumptive thrombocytopenia, microangiopathic hemolytic anemia, and organ dysfunction. The classic pentad where thrombocytopenia and hemolytic anemia are accompanied by fever, neurologic signs, and renal dysfunction, is observed only in a minority of patients. TTP remains a clinical diagnosis requiring exclusion of other causes of thrombotic microangiopathy such as DIC and severe hypertension.[60] Treatment of TTP is considered a medical emergency, and TPE should be initiated immediately. TPE with plasma-based fluid replacement has decreased the mortality from over 90% to between 10% and 20% (ASFA indication Category I[58]). If TPE is not readily available, infusion of plasma should be initiated (40 mL/kg or as the patient tolerates volume) until apheresis therapy can be arranged.

The majority of adult-onset cases of TTP have severe ADAMTS13 deficiency, attributable to inhibitory autoantibody. Absence or delay in determination of ADAMTS13 deficiency should not be the sole reason to withhold apheresis therapy.[60] Emerging consensus is that severe ADAMTS13 deficiency (<5 to 10% activity) distinguishes the more classic autoimmune idiopathic TTP from other forms of the syndrome; however, some of the ADAMTS13 nondeficient or moderately deficient presentations may still benefit from TPE. Along this line of reasoning, sufficient evidence has accumulated for several thrombotic microangiopathic syndromes, such as allogeneic progenitor cell transplantation and some drug-induced forms, where TPE is no longer recommended (see Chapter 7: Therapeutic Apheresis). Relapses are common, particularly with patients presenting with severe ADAMTS13 deficiency with inhibitors. The role for immunotherapy to prevent recurrences in acquired cases remains to be defined.[61] Congenital deficiency of the metalloprotease ADAMTS13 is a rare condition associated with congenital relapsing TTP where prophylactic plasma infusion may be useful in disease management.

Disorders of Fibrinolysis

Primary disorders of fibrinolysis are rare and hard to differentiate from DIC. Most fibrinolytic states are secondary to strong procoagulant stimuli. Antifibrinolytic therapy (eg, EACA) has been reported to be successful in the treatment of surgical settings where bleeding is attributable to activation of the fibrinolytic mechanism, such as cardiopulmonary bypass procedures and liver transplantation. However, the use of systemic EACA in other clinical settings may require a hematology consultation, because blockade of the fibrinolytic system can be associated with pathologic thrombosis.[44]

The therapeutic administration of the plasminogen activators streptokinase and urokinase or of recombinant tissue-type plasminogen activator has grown increasingly important in the treatment of thrombotic disease. These agents may be used locally (ie, infused via angiographic control directly into the thrombosed area) or systemically (ie, infused via the peripheral vein). Successful results have been reported in coronary and peripheral arterial disease as well as in venous thrombotic disorders. Contraindications to thrombolytic therapy include recent cranial trauma or known intracranial lesions and recent major surgery. Laboratory monitoring is not precise, and treatment regimens are standardized for each agent. The lytic state can be monitored by periodic assay of fibrinogen concentration or TT. Discontinuation of the drug and repletion of fibrinogen with Cryoprecipitated AHF are useful if a patient develops uncontrolled bleeding while receiving thrombolytic agents. Inhibitors of fibrinolysis should be used with extreme caution in this setting.

References

1. Slichter SJ. Evidence-based platelet transfusion guidelines. Hematology Am Soc Hematol Educ Program. 2007:172-8.
2. British Committee for Haematology. Blood transfusion: Guidelines for the use of platelet transfusion. Br J Haematol 2003;122:10-23.
3. Kuter DJ. General aspects of thrombocytopenia, platelet transfusions, and thrombopoietic growth factors. In: Kitch-

ens CS, Alving BM, Kessler CM, eds. Consultative hemostasis and thrombosis. 2nd ed. Philadelphia: Saunders Elsevier 2007:111-22.

4. Ferraris VA, Brown JR, Despotis GJ, et al. 2011 update to the Society of Thoracic Surgeons and the Society of Cardiovascular Anesthesiologists blood conservation clinical practice guidelines. Ann Thorac Surg 2011;91:944-82.

5. Brass L. Understanding and evaluating platelet function. Hematology Am Soc Hematol Educ Program 2010;387-96.

6. Kessler CM, Khokhar N, Liu M. A systematic approach to the bleeding patient. In: Kitchens CS, Alving BM, Kessler CM, eds. Consultative hemostasis and thrombosis. 2nd ed. Philadelphia: Saunders Elsevier 2007:17-34.

7. Chew DP, Moliterno DJ. A critical appraisal of platelet glycoprotein IIb/IIIa inhibition. J Am Coll Cardiol 2000;36:2028-35.

8. Becker RC. Hemostatic aspects of cardiovascular medicine. In: Kitchens CS, Alving BM, Kessler CM, eds. Consultative hemostasis and thrombosis. 2nd ed. Philadelphia: Saunders Elsevier 2007:339-69.

9. Curtis BR, Divgi A, Garritty M, Aster RH. Delayed thrombocytopenia after treatment with abciximab: A distinct clinical entity associated with the immune response to the drug. J Thromb Haemost 2004;2:985-92.

10. Furie B, Furie BC. In vivo thrombus formation. J Thromb Haemost 2007;5 (Suppl 1):12-17.

11. British Committee for Standards in Haematology Transfusion Task Force. Guidelines for the use of fresh frozen plasma, cryoprecipitate, and cryosupernatant. Br J Haematol 2004;126:11-28.

12. Senzolo M, Burroughs AK. Hemostatic alterations in liver disease and liver transplantation. In: Kitchens CS, Alving BM, Kessler CM, eds. Consultative hemostasis and thrombosis. 2nd ed. Philadelphia: Saunders Elsevier 2007:647-59.

13. Segal JB, Dzik WH. Paucity of studies to support that abnormal coagulation test results predict bleeding in the

setting of invasive procedures: An evidence-based review. Transfusion 2005;45:1413-25.

14. Roberts HR, Escobar MA. Less common congenital disorders of hemostasis. In: Kitchens CS, Alving BM, Kessler CM, eds. Consultative hemostasis and thrombosis. 2nd ed. Philadelphia: Saunders Elsevier 2007:61-80.

15. Boggio LN, Kessler CM. Hemophilia A and B. In: Kitchens CS, Alving BM, Kessler CM, eds. Consultative hemostasis and thrombosis. 2nd ed. Philadelphia: Saunders Elsevier 2007:45-60.

16. DeLoughery TG. Logistics of massive transfusions. Hematology Am Soc Hematol Educ Program 2010:470-3.

17. Heit JA. Thrombophilia: Common questions on laboratory assessment and management. Hematology Am Soc Hematol Educ Program 2007:127-35.

18. Bauer KA. Duration of anticoagulation: Applying the guidelines and beyond. Hematology Am Soc Hematol Educ Program 2010:210-15.

19. Abshire TC. Laboratory assessment of fibrinolysis. In: Hillyer CD, Shaz BH, Zimring JC, Abshire TC, eds. Transfusion medicine and hemostasis: Clinical and laboratory aspects. Burlington, MA: Elsevier 2009:671-75.

20. Enriquez LJ, Shore-Lesserson L. Point-of-care coagulation testing and transfusion algorithms. Br J Anaesth 2009;103 (Suppl 1):i14-i22.

21. Neunert C, Lim W, Crowther M, et al. The American Society of Hematology 2011 evidence-based practice guideline for immune thrombocytopenia. Blood 2011;117:4190-207.

22. Warkentin TE, Greinacher A, Koster A, Lincoff AM. Treatment and prevention of heparin-induced thrombocytopenia: American College of Chest Physicians evidence-based clinical practice guidelines (8th ed). Chest 2008; 133:340S-380S.

23. Swisher KK, Terrell DR, Vesely SK et al. Clinical outcomes after platelet transfusions in patients with thrombotic thrombocytopenic purpura. Transfusion 2009;49:873-87.

24. Jobe S, Di Paola J. Congenital and acquired disorders of platelet function and number. In: Kitchens CS, Alving BM, Kessler CM, eds. Consultative hemostasis and thrombosis. 2nd ed. Philadelphia: Saunders Elsevier 2007:139-58.

25. Bolton-Maggs PH, Chalmers EA, Collins PW, et al. A review of inherited platelet disorders with guidelines for their management on behalf of the UKHCDO. Br J Haematol 2006;135:603-33.

26. Nichols WL, Hultin MB, James AH, et al. von Willebrand disease (VWD): Evidence-based diagnosis and management guidelines, the National Heart, Lung, and Blood Institute (NHLBI) Expert Panel report (USA). Haemophilia 2008;14:171-232.

27. Bolan CD, Klein HG. Blood component and pharmacologic therapy of hemostatic disorders. In: Kitchens CS, Alving BM, Kessler CM, eds. Consultative hemostasis and thrombosis. 2nd ed. Philadelphia: Saunders Elsevier 2007:461-90.

28. Serrano K, Scammell K, Weiss S, et al. Plasma and cryoprecipitate manufactured from whole blood held overnight at room temperature meet quality standards. Transfusion 2010;50:344-53.

29. Dunn AL, Abshire TC. Recent advances in the management of the child who has hemophilia. Hematol Oncol Clin North Am 2004;18:1249-76, viii.

30. Batorova A, Martinowitz U. Continuous infusion of coagulation factors: Current opinion. Curr Opin Hematol 2006; 13:308-15.

31. Hay CR, Brown S, Collins PW, et al. The diagnosis and management of factor VIII and IX inhibitors: A guideline from the United Kingdom Haemophilia Centre Doctors Organisation. Br J Haematol 2006;133:591-605.

32. Levi M, Levy JH, Andersen HF, Truloff D. Safety of recombinant activated factor VII in randomized clinical trials. N Engl J Med 2010;363:1791-800.

33. Gomez K, Bolton-Maggs P. Factor XI deficiency. Haemophilia 2008;14:1183-9.

34. Lapecorella M, Mariani G. Factor VII deficiency: Defining the clinical picture and optimizing therapeutic options. Haemophilia 2008;14:1170-5.

35. Scott E, Puca K, Heraly J, et al. Evaluation and comparison of coagulation factor activity in fresh-frozen plasma and 24-hour plasma at thaw and after 120 hours of 1 to 6 degrees C storage. Transfusion 2009;49:1584-91.

36. Yazer MH, Cortese-Hassett A, Triulzi DJ. Coagulation factor levels in plasma frozen within 24 hours of phlebotomy over 5 days of storage at 1 to 6 degrees C. Transfusion 2008;48:2525-30.

37. Hsieh L, Nugent D. Factor XIII deficiency. Haemophilia 2008;14:1190-200.

38. Acharya SS, Dimichele DM. Rare inherited disorders of fibrinogen. Haemophilia 2008;14:1151-8.

39. Favier R, Aoki N, de Moerloose P. Congenital alpha(2)-plasmin inhibitor deficiencies: A review. Br J Haematol 2001;114:4-10.

40. Schulman S, Bijsterveld NR. Anticoagulants and their reversal. Transfus Med Rev 2007;21:37-48.

41. Holland L, Warkentin TE, Refaai M, et al. Suboptimal effect of a three-factor prothrombin complex concentrate (Profilnine-SD) in correcting supratherapeutic international normalized ratio due to warfarin overdose. Transfusion 2009;49:1171-7.

42. Logan AC, Goodnough LT. Recombinant factor VIIa: An assessment of evidence regarding its efficacy and safety in the off-label setting. Hematology Am Soc Hematol Educ Program 2010:153-9.

43. Levi M. Disseminated intravascular coagulation. Crit Care Med 2007;35:2191-5.

44. Levi M, Toh CH, Thachil J, Watson HG. Guidelines for the diagnosis and management of disseminated intravascular coagulation. British Committee for Standards in Haematology. Br J Haematol 2009;145:24-33.

45. Holcomb JB. Optimal use of blood products in severely injured trauma patients. Hematology Am Soc Hematol Educ Program 2010:465-9.
46. Zimrin AB, Holcomb JB, Hess JR. Hemorrhage control and thrombosis following severe injury. In: Kitchens CS, Alving BM, Kessler CM, eds. Consultative hemostasis and thrombosis. 2nd ed. Philadelphia: Saunders Elsevier 2007: 717-22.
47. Schulman S, Beyth RJ, Kearon C, Levine MN. Hemorrhagic complications of anticoagulant and thrombolytic treatment: American College of Chest Physicians evidence-based clinical practice guidelines (8th ed). Chest 2008;133:257S-298S.
48. Di NM, Middeldorp S, Buller HR. Direct thrombin inhibitors. N Engl J Med 2005;353:1028-40.
49. van Ryn J, Stangier J, Haertter S, et al. Dabigatran etexilate—a novel, reversible, oral direct thrombin inhibitor: Interpretation of coagulation assays and reversal of anticoagulant activity. Thromb Haemost 2010;103:1116-27.
50. Douketis JD. Pharmacologic properties of the new oral anticoagulants: A clinician-oriented review with a focus on perioperative management. Curr Pharm Des 2010;16:3436-41.
51. Messmore HL Jr., Jeske WP, Wehrmacher W, et al. Antiplatelet agents: Current drugs and future trends. Hematol Oncol Clin North Am 2005;19:87-117,vi.
52. Bates SM, Greer IA, Pabinger I, et al. Venous thromboembolism, thrombophilia, antithrombotic therapy, and pregnancy: American College of Chest Physicians evidence-based clinical practice guidelines (8th ed). Chest 2008;133: 844S-886S.
53. Rodger M. Evidence base for the management of venous thromboembolism in pregnancy. Hematology Am Soc Hematol Educ Program 2010:173-80.
54. Patnaik MM, Moll S. Inherited antithrombin deficiency: A review. Haemophilia 2008;14:1229-39.

55. Heit JA. Thrombophilia: Clinical and laboratory assessment and management. In: Kitchens CS, Alving BM, Kessler CM, eds. Consultative hemostasis and thrombosis. 2nd ed. Philadelphia: Saunders Elsevier, 2007:213-44.

56. Goldenberg NA, Manco-Johnson MJ. Protein C deficiency. Haemophilia 2008;14:1214-21.

57. Rand JH. The antiphospholipid syndrome: Clinical presentation, diagnosis, and patient management. In: Kitchens CS, Alving BM, Kessler CM, eds. Consultative hemostasis and thrombosis. 2nd ed. Philadelphia: Saunders Elsevier, 2007:338.

58. Szczepiorkowski ZM, Winters JL, Bandarenko N, et al. Guidelines on the use of therapeutic apheresis in clinical practice—evidence-based approach from the Apheresis Applications Committee of the American Society for Apheresis. J Clin Apher 2010;25:83-177.

59. Raflores MB, Kaplan RB, Spero JA. Pre-operative management of a patient with hypoprothrombinemia-lupus anticoagulant syndrome. Thromb Haemost 2007;98:248-50.

60. Greinacher A, Selleng K. Thrombocytopenia in the intensive care unit patient. Hematology Am Soc Hematol Educ Program 2010:135-43.

61. Peyvandi F, Palla R, Lotta LA. Pathogenesis and treatment of acquired idiopathic thrombotic thrombocytopenic purpura. Haematologica 2010;95:1444-7.

ADVERSE EFFECTS OF BLOOD TRANSFUSION

Because of the risk of adverse reactions, transfusion should be administered only when the benefits clearly outweigh the risks. Patients should be advised of the risks, benefits, and alternatives to transfusion and of the consequences of refusal of transfusion. Documentation of patient consent is required. All suspected transfusion reactions should be reported to the transfusion service for investigation and guidance on further recommendations for component therapy.

Acute Transfusion Reactions

Acute transfusion reactions occur during or within 24 hours after a transfusion. Most life-threatening transfusion reactions occur early in the course of transfusion; therefore, all patients should be monitored carefully throughout transfusion, and any adverse signs and symptoms should be investigated promptly. If a reaction occurs during the course of a multiple-unit transfusion, the unit currently being transfused may not necessarily be the cause of the reaction.

Acute Hemolytic Reactions

Hemolytic transfusion reactions (HTRs) are caused by immune-mediated lysis of transfused red cells. Such reactions can be acute or delayed and can result in intravascular or extravascular hemolysis. An acute HTR (AHTR) occurs when incompatible red cells are transfused to a recipient who already has a clinically significant antibody to an antigen present on the transfused cells, as in the transfusion of group A red cells to a group O or a group B recipient. Many fatal HTRs are the result of transfusion of ABO-incompatible blood; however, fatal HTRs caused by other blood group antibodies do occur. During fiscal years 2005, 2006, and 2009 more fatal HTRs caused by non-ABO blood group antibodies were reported to the Food and Drug Administration (FDA) than those caused by ABO incompatibility.[1] Patient misidentification during patient sample collection, compatibility testing, or blood administration is the most common cause of ABO-incompatibility-induced acute hemolysis. HTRs typically occur within minutes of the start of the infusion. If the recipient's antibody fixes complement, as most often occurs with ABO-incompatible blood transfusions, an acute intravascular HTR results.[2] The anti-A and anti-B responsible are either IgM or complement-fixing IgG, which results in the binding of the C5b-9 component of complement (the membrane attack complex). Fixation of C5b-9 results in a pore in the red cell membrane. Water enters the cell through this pore, and osmotic intravascular lysis results, which produces hemoglobinemia. This can result in an increase of plasma hemoglobin to 200 mg/dL or more, which will lend plasma a pink to red color. If the plasma hemoglobin is only moderately increased, between 10 and 40 mg/dL, plasma discoloration may be less evident due to other pigments such as bilirubin (yellow) or methemalbumin (brown). The renal glomerulus filters free hemoglobin molecules once plasma haptoglobin is saturated; this results in hemoglobinuria.[3] These two signs are critical for the diagnosis of an AHTR. Characteristic laboratory findings may also include decreased hematocrit, decreased haptoglobin, increased lactate dehydrogenase (LDH), and the presence of plasma hemoglobin. Serum bilirubin typically increases 6 to 12 hours later.

The severe clinical symptoms of shock and hypotension seen in an AHTR are caused by the generated complement fragments, anaphylatoxins C3a and C5a, and other mediators of inflammation.[2-3] In addition, hypotension can lead to renal ischemia, which may result in tubular necrosis and the development of acute renal failure. The binding of nitric oxide by free hemoglobin exacerbates renal ischemia. Nitric oxide is a potent vasodilator. Nitric oxide activity is balanced by endothelin, a potent vasoconstrictor. Hemoglobin scavenging of nitric oxide thus promotes renal vasoconstriction, tubular necrosis, and renal failure.[4] The coagulation cascade may be activated as well, initiating disseminated intravascular coagulation (DIC). Clinical symptoms are in large part attributable to activation of the cytokine network, including the proinflammatory cytokines interleukin-1 (IL-1), IL-6, IL-8, and tumor necrosis factor-alpha (TNF-α), which produce fever, hypotension, and activation of white cells and the clotting cascade.[5,6]

The severity of an AHTR depends on the rate and amount of blood transfused. Generally, a larger volume of incompatible blood transfused and a faster infusion rate result in a more severe reaction. Treatment of an AHTR, a medical emergency, is described in Table 6. If an AHTR is suspected, infusion of the unit should be stopped immediately, and additional Red Blood Cell (RBC) units should not be administered until the cause has been identified and corrected. When transfusion is urgent, communication with the blood bank is critical. The occurrence of acute intravascular hemolysis in the absence of red cell incompatibility should prompt the search for a nonimmunologic cause of the hemolysis (see below).

Whereas most AHTRs are intravascular, if the antibody does not fix complement or fixes only to C3, the resulting reaction will be an acute extravascular HTR (Table 7). Acute extravascular HTRs are not associated with the serious clinical symptom complex seen in acute intravascular HTRs, because extravascular HTRs involve much less generation of proinflammatory cytokines.[7] Acute extravascular HTRs typically present with fever, a positive direct antiglobulin test (DAT or Coombs test) caused by antibody binding to the transfused incompatible red cells, and a decreasing hematocrit without any overt signs of bleeding. Hemoglobinemia and hemoglobinuria are rarely seen. Severe

Table 6. Workup of an Acute Transfusion Reaction

If an acute transfusion reaction occurs:

1. Stop blood component transfusion immediately.

2. Verify the correct unit was given to the correct patient.

3. Maintain IV access and ensure adequate urine output with an appropriate crystalloid or colloid solution.

4. Maintain blood pressure and pulse.

5. Maintain adequate ventilation.

6. Notify attending physician and blood bank.

7. Obtain blood/urine for transfusion reaction workup.

8. Send report of reaction, samples, blood bag, and administration set to blood bank.

9. Blood bank performs workup of suspected transfusion reaction as follows:

   A. A clerical check is performed to ensure correct blood component was transfused to the right patient.

   B. The plasma is visually evaluated for hemoglobinemia.

   C. A direct antiglobulin test is performed.

   D. Other serologic testing is repeated as needed (ABO, Rh, crossmatch).

If an intravascular hemolytic reaction is confirmed:

1. Monitor renal status (BUN, creatinine).

2. Initiate diuresis; avoid fluid overload if renal failure is present.

3. Analyze urine for hemoglobinuria.

4. Monitor coagulation status (PT, aPTT, fibrinogen, platelet count).

5. Monitor for signs of hemolysis (LDH, bilirubin, haptoglobin, plasma hemoglobin).

6. Monitor hemoglobin and hematocrit.

7. Repeat compatibility testing (crossmatch).

8. **Consult with blood bank physician before further transfusion.**

Table 6. Workup of an Acute Transfusion Reaction (Continued)

If bacterial contamination is suspected:

1. Obtain blood culture of patient.

2. Return unit or empty blood bag to blood bank for culture and Gram's stain.

3. Maintain circulation and urine output.

4. Initiate broad-spectrum antibiotic treatment as appropriate; revise antibiotic regimen on the basis of microbiological results.

5. Monitor for signs of DIC, renal failure, respiratory failure.

IV = intravenous; BUN = blood urea nitrogen; PT = prothrombin time; aPTT = activated partial thromboplastin time; LDH = lactate dehydrogenase; DIC = disseminated intravascular coagulation. Adapted from Wu Y, Mantha S, Snyder EL. Transfusion reactions. In: Hoffman R, Benz EF Jr, Shattil SJ, et al. Hematology: Basic principles and practice. 5th ed. New York: Churchill Livingstone, 2008:2267-75.

hemolytic reactions may also occur in association with the infusion of incompatible plasma, which may occur with transfusion of ABO-incompatible platelets (such as group O platelets to a group A patient) and, rarely, with that of intravenous immune globulin (IVIG) or intermediate-purity Factor VIII concentrates.[8-10]

Sickle Cell Hemolytic Transfusion Reaction Syndrome

Multitransfused patients with sickle cell disease have a greater incidence of red cell alloimmunization because of frequent transfusion and red cell phenotype differences from the general donor population. HTRs in sickle cell disease can precipitate a hemolytic crisis and result in a greater degree of anemia than before transfusion because of bystander hemolysis of autologous red cells and/or the sickle cell HTR syndrome.[11,12] In this syndrome, there is a suppression of endogenous erythropoiesis and a

Table 7. Acute Transfusion Reactions

Type	Signs and Symptoms	Usual Cause	Treatment	Prevention
Intravascular hemolytic (immune)	Hemoglobinemia and hemoglobinuria, fever, chills, anxiety, shock, DIC, dyspnea, chest pain, flank pain, oliguria	ABO incompatibility (clerical error) or other complement-fixing red cell antibody	Stop transfusion; hydrate, support blood pressure and respiration; induce diuresis; treat shock and DIC, if present	Ensure proper sample and recipient identification
Extravascular hemolytic (immune)	Fever, malaise, indirect hyperbilirubinemia, increased LDH, urine urobilinogen, falling hematocrit	IgG non-complement-fixing antibody	Monitor hematocrit, renal and hepatic function, coagulation profile; no acute treatment generally required	Review historical records; ensure proper sample and recipient identification; give antigen-negative units as appropriate; possible high-dose IVIG

Febrile	Fever, chills	Antibodies to leukocytes or plasma proteins; hemolysis; passive cytokine infusion; bacterial contamination; commonly due to patient's underlying condition	Stop transfusion; give antipyretics, eg, acetaminophen; for rigors in adults, use meperidine 25 to 50 mg IV or IM	Pretransfusion antipyretic; leukocyte-reduced blood components
Allergic (mild to severe)	Urticaria (hives), dyspnea, wheezing, throat tightening; rarely, hypotension or anaphylaxis	Antibodies to plasma proteins; rarely, antibodies to IgA	Stop transfusion; give antihistamine (PO or IM); if severe, epinephrine and/or steroids	Pretransfusion antihistamine; washed red cells, if recurrent or severe; check pretransfusion IgA levels in patients with a history of anaphylaxis to transfusion

(Continued)

Table 7. Acute Transfusion Reactions (Continued)

Type	Signs and Symptoms	Usual Cause	Treatment	Prevention
Circulatory overload	Dyspnea, hypertension, pulmonary edema, cardiac arrhythmias	Too rapid and/or excessive blood transfusion volume	Induce diuresis; phlebotomy; support cardiorespiratory system as needed	Avoid rapid or excessive transfusion volume
Transfusion-related acute lung injury (TRALI)	Dyspnea, fever, hypoxia, pulmonary edema, hypotension, normal pulmonary capillary wedge pressure	Donor HLA or leukocyte antibody transfused with plasma in component; neutrophil-priming lipid mediator; less commonly, recipient antibody to donor white cells	Support blood pressure and respiration (may require intubation)	Leukocyte-reduced red cells and platelets; notify transfusion service and blood center to test donor(s); quarantine remaining components from donor(s)

| Hypotension | Hypotension, tachycardia | Bradykinin generation; may be exacerbated by ACE inhibitor | Stop transfusion; give fluids; use Trendelenberg position | Discontinue ACE inhibitor; avoid bedside leukocyte-reduction filters |
| Bacterial contamination | Rigors, chills, fever, shock | Contaminated blood component | Stop transfusion; support blood pressure; culture patient and blood unit; give antibiotics; notify blood transfusion service | Care in donor selection, blood collection and storage; careful attention to arm preparation for phlebotomy |

DIC = disseminated intravascular coagulation; IV = intravenous; IM = intramuscular; PO = by mouth; ACE = angiotensin-converting enzyme; LDH = lactate dehydrogenase; IVIG = intravenous immune globulin; IgA = immunoglobulin A.

decrease in the absolute number of HbS-containing red cells.[11,12] Painful crisis in a patient with sickle cell disease after transfusion should suggest the occurrence of sickle cell HTR syndrome. Further transfusion in the setting of bystander hemolysis or sickle cell HTR syndrome may exacerbate the anemia, and may even prove fatal. Therefore, the decision to transfuse RBCs must be carefully measured with consideration given to the fact that not transfusing may be most helpful. Iatrogenic blood loss should be avoided. To avoid additional transfusion in this setting, corticosteroids and erythropoietin are often administered as is IVIG.[13,14] Serologic studies may not provide a clear explanation for HTRs in these patients, in part because the presence of multiple alloantibodies may make the serologic diagnosis difficult. On the other hand, alloantibodies may not be detected at all; in these patients the mechanism may be related to the induction of phosphatidylserine exposure on donor red cells, which leads to accelerated donor red cell destruction that eventually leads to autologous red cell destruction as well.[15]

Drug-Induced Hemolysis

Many drugs can induce the production of antibodies against red cells and cause hemolysis. Whereas drug-induced hemolysis is not a transfusion reaction, it can be readily confused with an HTR in the transfused patient. In drug-induced hemolysis, both autologous and transfused red cells will be eliminated. Typically, there is a positive DAT result, and the serum will react with red cells in the presence, but not the absence, of the offending drug. Clinically, drug-induced hemolysis may be indistinguishable from an HTR. The hemolysis may be severe and even fatal. Treatment consists of discontinuing the drug, providing supportive care, and administering transfusion to maintain adequate oxygen-carrying capacity. Cefotetan and ceftriaxone are among the most common causes of drug-induced hemolysis; however, nonsteroidal anti-inflammatory drugs should not be overlooked.[16]

Nonimmune Hemolysis

Mechanical hemolysis of transfused blood, caused by shear stress imposed on erythrocytes, can occur with artificial heart valves, with extracorporeal circulation, or with transfusion through small-bore catheters under high pressure. Administration of hypotonic saline solutions, 5% dextrose in water, distilled water, or certain medications in the same line as the blood infusion can result in osmotic lysis of transfused red cells. Heating above 42 C that results from a malfunction of the blood warmer or freezing because of exposure to ice or a refrigerator malfunction may hemolyze blood before transfusion. Hemoglobinuria may occur in nonimmune hemolysis. Transfusion of hemolyzed blood can cause hyperkalemia and transient renal impairment. The cause of hemoglobinemia and/or hemoglobinuria must be evaluated as soon as possible, because delay in the recognition of an immune HTR could lead to serious clinical complications.

Febrile Nonhemolytic Transfusion Reactions

Fever is a common sign of a transfusion reaction (Table 7) and may be the first sign of a febrile reaction, bacterial contamination, or an AHTR. Fever results from the production of pyrogens (IL-1, IL-6, and TNF-α) that act on the thermoregulatory center in the hypothalamus through the intermediary of prostaglandin E2. Fever may be caused by the patient's underlying condition; thus fever, per se, is not a contraindication for administering a blood transfusion. A febrile nonhemolytic transfusion reaction (FNHTR) is defined as occurring during or within 4 hours of transfusion and either a fever greater than 38 C orally and an increase of ≥ 1 C from the pretransfusion temperature, or chills/rigors. A FNHTR may occur without a measured fever if chills and/or rigors are the only presenting symptoms. Febrile reactions may be attributed to antibodies directed against transfused leukocytes or platelets. The resulting antigen-antibody reactions trigger phagocytes to release endogenous pyrogens, which causes fever.[5,17] Alternatively, leukocytes in cellular blood components may produce pyrogens during storage.[18] The use of leukocyte-reduced blood components can mitigate, but not necessarily eliminate, these reactions.[19,20]

Pyrogenic cytokines may be produced by events that are unrelated to the transfusion. The diagnosis of FNHTR is therefore one of exclusion. Transfusion of stored blood components containing preformed cytokines may explain why some patients experience FNHTRs despite bedside filtration. Prestorage leukocyte reduction can reduce the accumulation of pyrogens.[21] The incidence of FNHTRs with red cells has been reported between 0.04 and 0.44 per 100 units. The incidence with platelets ranges from 0.06 to 2.2 reactions per 100 transfusions. A higher incidence is seen when components are not leukocyte reduced before storage.[18,22] Another postulated mechanism for FNHTRs is that, during storage, platelets also release CD40 ligand (CD154), which can stimulate endothelial cells to produce prostaglandin E2 in a manner similar to pyrogenic cytokines.[23]

Most FNHTRs respond to treatment with antipyretics. In general, aspirin should not be used in thrombocytopenic patients. For such patients, acetaminophen or nonsteroidal anti-inflammatory agents are preferred. Acetaminophen has commonly been prescribed for prophylaxis; however, the evidence supporting efficacy of this practice is questionable.[24] FNHTRs are rarely serious, but rigors can be a significant stress for a patient with compromised cardiorespiratory status. Rigors may be treated with opioids, although they should be used with caution in patients with impaired respiratory drive. Antihistamines do not prevent febrile reactions and have no role in prophylaxis.

Allergic Reactions

Allergic reactions occur in about 1% to 3% of all transfusion recipients. Most allergic reactions are mild, and are limited to pruritis, urticaria, and flushing.[25] With mild, localized reactions, the transfusion may be continued under observation after oral or parenteral antihistamines are given, provided the signs and symptoms subside. It should be stressed that this possibility applies only to mild allergic transfusion reactions and not to severe reactions in patients presenting with fever, chills, dyspnea, wheezing, or laryngeal edema, which would warrant investigation by the transfusion service and treatment of an anaphylactic reaction, which is rare. Readers should refer to their own institutional policies on reporting allergic reactions.

Anaphylactic reactions can be caused by antibodies to IgA, haptoglobin, or C4 (Chido/Rodgers blood group antigens).[26-28] For severe allergic or anaphylactic reactions, the transfusion should be stopped immediately, and intravenous (IV) access should be secured while fluid resuscitation and treatment with epinephrine and/or steroids are started. Severe reactions may require treatment with vasopressors and intubation. When further transfusion is indicated, washed cellular blood components should be considered.[29] Transfusion of components containing plasma to such patients presents a difficult problem that requires a careful risk/benefit analysis. Pretransfusion treatment with high-dose corticosteroids, antihistamines, or H2-blockers should be considered, and the immediate availability of epinephrine should be ensured. A typical dose schedule is to medicate the patient 30 to 60 minutes before transfusion with 100 mg of hydrocortisone given intravenously and 25 to 50 mg of diphenhydramine given orally or parenterally. IgA-deficient patients may require IgA-deficient plasma that can be obtained through rare-donor registries.

Because allergic reactions are so common, diphenhydramine is often used as preventive premedication. However, in a prospective randomized study, this practice was not shown to decrease the rate of urticarial reactions.[30] Leukocyte reduction of components does not prevent allergic reactions.

Circulatory Overload

Transfusion-associated circulatory overload (TACO) develops when the patient is unable to compensate for expanded blood volume. Signs and symptoms of TACO include headache, shortness of breath, pulmonary edema, congestive heart failure, and systolic hypertension (>50 mm Hg increase). B-type natriuretic peptide (BNP) can be useful in distinguishing TACO from other causes. Symptoms usually subside if the transfusion is stopped, and the patient is placed in a sitting position and given oxygen and diuretics to remove fluid. If symptoms persist, a phlebotomy may be necessary.[31] Rarely, hypertension with volume overload can lead to flash pulmonary edema. To avoid hypervolemia, blood components should not be infused at a rate faster than 2 to 4 mL/kg/hour. Slower rates are needed for patients at risk of TACO, such as patients with chronic anemia who have an expanded plasma volume or patients with compromised cardiac and/or pulmonary function. In these situations, a single or split unit of blood can be transfused slowly over time, not to exceed 4 hours.

Transfusion-Related Acute Lung Injury

Dyspnea, fever, chills, hypotension, and new onset bilateral pulmonary edema associated with transfusion may indicate transfusion-related acute lung injury (TRALI). TRALI has been defined as acute lung injury with hypoxemia and $PaO_2/FiO_2 \leq 300$ or $SpO_2 < 90\%$ on room air, where there were no prior risk factors for acute lung injury before transfusion, with the onset of symptoms within 6 hours of transfusion.[32] It is differentiated from TACO by the lack of left atrial hypertension, nonelevated BNP levels, and unresponsiveness to diuresis.[32,33] The infusion of HLA- or granulocyte-specific antibody in plasma-containing components, which then reacts with a recipient antigen, is hypothesized as the most common cause of this reaction. The donor of the implicated unit is often a multiparous woman.[34] Less commonly, recipient antibodies directed against donor leukocytes are implicated as a cause of TRALI. Alternatively, oxidation of membrane lipids produced by donor leukocytes during storage may prime recipient neutrophils so that a second stimulus, such as inflammation, infection, or tissue injury, results in the release of vasoactive mediators (the two-hit hypothesis).[35] Recipient factors may also determine susceptibility to TRALI because, in look-back cases, not all recipients of blood from an implicated donor manifest TRALI, even when there is HLA antibody-antigen concordance.[36,37]

In its full form, TRALI presents most commonly within 2 to 6 hours of a transfusion as marked respiratory distress, hypoxia, hypotension, fever, and bilateral pulmonary edema.[32,33] However, milder forms of TRALI may be difficult to recognize as such. TRALI reactions typically resolve within 48 to 72 hours, although the mortality rate is approximately 10%. In most instances no special requirements are necessary to manage further transfusions; however, leukocyte-reduced components are indicated for subsequent transfusions if the reaction was caused by recipient HLA antibodies. The treatment of TRALI reactions is supportive. The patient may require supplemental oxygen, endotracheal intubation, and respiratory support until the intra-alveolar fluid can be resorbed. Diuresis is not indicated. The role of steroids in therapy is not clear. Fluid support may be necessary for resuscitation in the event of hypotension and marked movement of fluid from plasma to the extravascular space. Suspected TRALI reactions should be reported to the blood supplier immediately to ascertain information about the donor(s) of the transfused blood components and to allow the quarantine or recall of additional components from the donor(s). A test for HLA and granulocyte antibodies in donor plasma—and, if that test is positive, HLA and granulocyte antigen typing of the recipient—may help establish the diagnosis. Because TRALI is one of the most common causes of transfusion-associated mortality in the United States and fatal reactions have been linked to components produced from multiparous female donors, many blood suppliers are no longer producing plasma from these donors in order to decrease the risk of TRALI.[38] In addition, apheresis platelet donors are now also screened for HLA antibodies.

Hypotensive Reactions to Transfusion

Hypotensive reactions following platelet and red cell transfusions have been reported. These reactions are defined as a drop in systolic and/or diastolic blood pressure of more than 30 mm Hg in adults, and for infants or children a decrease of more than 25% from the baseline blood pressure. To be considered transfusion associated, the hypotension should occur during or within 1 hour of transfusion, and may also be seen with facial flushing, dyspnea, or abdominal cramps. However, in most cases hypotension is the sole manifestation. These reactions appear to involve the generation of bradykinin from activation of the kinin pathway caused by contact of plasma with artificial surfaces. Bradykinin is a potent vasodilator that causes hypotension, abdominal pain, and facial flushing.[39-41] Some of these reactions have occurred in patients receiving blood through a negatively charged bedside leukocyte reduction filter while they were medicated with angiotensin-converting enzyme (ACE) inhibitor drugs. ACE is identical to kininase II, the principal enzyme that degrades bradykinin. The inhibition of kininase II prolongs the half-life of bradykinin in these patients and can worsen the clinical symptoms. Because bradykinin has a half-life of 15 to 30 seconds, prestorage leukocyte reduction rather than bedside leukocyte reduction should eliminate reactions caused by contact with the filter biomaterials. Transfusion-associated hypotension typically resolves within minutes of the cessation of the transfusion. Whenever such reactions occur, they must be differentiated from vasovagal reactions, TRALI, HTRs, bacterial contamination, anaphylaxis, and the patient's underlying medical condition. This is best accomplished by reporting these reactions to the transfusion service for investigation.

Bacterial Contamination

Bacterial contamination of stored blood poses a rare but serious risk to the transfusion recipient. Bacteria can enter a blood bag because of improper preparation of the skin at the venipuncture site at the time of phlebotomy, during component preparation or handling, during shipping, or because of occult bacteremia in the donor. The overall rate of bacterial contamination of blood collections determined by prospective culture has been reported to be as high as 0.3%, although the incidence of serious reactions is less (see Table 8). Skin flora (ie, *Staphylococcus* and *Propionibacteria*) are the most common isolates from prospectively cultured units, but other species are more often implicated in clinical reactions. Gram-negative rods (ie, *Acinetobacter, Klebsiella*, and *Escherichia*) are more common than gram-positive cocci (ie, *Staphylococcus* and *Streptococcus*) in fatal reactions to contaminated RBC and Platelet units.[42,43] Bacteria such as *Yersinia* or *Pseudomonas*, which are capable of growing at low tem-

Table 8. Bacterial Contamination Cases (Fatalities) Reported in the United States (1998-2000)

Organism	No. of Cases
Gram positive	
Bacillus cereus	1
Coagulase-negative *Staphylococci*	9
Streptococcus sp.	3 (1)
Staphylococcus aureus	4
Subtotal	17 (1 = 6%)*
Gram negative	
Serratia sp.	2 (2)
Escherichia coli	5 (1)
Enterobacter sp.	2 (1)
Providencia rettgeri	1 (1)
Yersinia enterocolitica	1
Subtotal	11 (5 = 45%)
Total	28 (6 = 21%)

*There were 17 cases of gram-positive organisms identified; however, only one case (1/17 = 6%) resulted in a fatality. Data from Kuehnert MJ, Roth VR, Haley NR, et al. Transfusion-transmitted bacterial infection in the United States, 1998 through 2000. Transfusion 2001;41:1493-9.

peratures in an iron-rich environment, may proliferate in RBC units. Although contaminated RBC units may appear dark or contain clots, visual inspection of components is not sensitive for detection of bacterial contamination of blood components.

During or after the transfusion, the patient *may* develop rigors, high fever, dyspnea, hypotension, and shock. Hemoglobinemia and hemoglobinuria are usually absent, and the posttransfusion DAT is usually negative. It is essential that any transfusion in progress be stopped when a contaminated unit is suspected. Aggressive resuscitative therapy and broad-spectrum antibiotics should be started immediately when a septic transfusion reaction is suspected. Additional components from the same donation, a common possibility with split apheresis components, could be infected and must be recalled. Therefore, suspected septic transfusion reactions should be reported immediately to the transfusion service and in turn to the blood collection center in order to prevent similar or even more severe reactions in other recipients. The suspected unit should be evaluated by the microbiology laboratory, and blood cultures should also be drawn from the patient. Septic reactions may not manifest until several hours after the transfusion of a unit of contaminated blood.

Adoption of methods to limit and detect bacterial contamination in platelet components[44] have decreased but not eliminated septic transfusion reactions. A study of over one million apheresis platelet donations prospectively screened by culture found 186 donations with positive cultures; transfusion of all but one was prevented. Products that screened negative were still implicated in 20 septic reactions, including three fatalities.[45]

Thermal Effects

The rapid transfusion of blood directly from refrigerator storage can result in hypothermia and resultant cardiac arrythmia or arrest. Conversely, overwarming blood can produce hemolysis. Blood should be warmed only by using an FDA-approved blood-warming device (see Chapter 3: Transfusion Practices). Warming blood with heating pads, hot tap water, or in a microwave oven is unacceptable.

Metabolic Complications

Blood is anticoagulated with citrate, which chelates calcium ions. If citrated blood is infused rapidly and the ionized calcium level decreases transiently, the patient may complain of tingling around the mouth (circumoral paresthesia) and in the fingers.[46] These symptoms subside quickly if the transfusion is slowed, because citrate is rapidly metabolized by patients with normal liver function. Under no circumstances should calcium be added to a unit of blood, because it could reverse the anticoagulant effect of the citrate, which would result in large blood clots.

During storage of red cells, there is reversible leakage of potassium into the supernatant. Although the potassium concentration may be high, the total amount of potassium in an RBC unit is usually inconsequential. Hyperkalemia caused by the massive infusion of stored blood is rare. Hyperkalemia may be a concern in neonates (especially in the context of exchange transfusion) and sometimes in liver transplantation, pediatric cardiac surgery, and in patients with renal failure. Washing of red cells, removal of the supernatant, or use of blood less than 7 days old can be helpful in such cases. If irradiation is required, it may be best to wash after irradiation is performed.[47] With large-volume transfusion, the production of bicarbonate from the infused citrate more often produces an alkalosis, which results in hypokalemia that may require potassium administration.[48]

Delayed Transfusion Reactions

Delayed Hemolytic Transfusion Reactions

Delayed HTRs (DHTRs) occur when the survival of transfused red cells is decreased after production of an alloantibody response in a recipient days or weeks after the transfusion episode. The difference in the time of antibody production relates to whether it is an anamnestic response (days) or a primary response (weeks) to transfusion. It has been estimated that, with each additional unit of blood transfused, there is a 2% to 6% risk of immunizing a recipient to a red cell antigen other than the D antigen.[49] Most DHTRs are extravascular, and they are often associated with antibodies to Rh and Kell system antigens. Because the antibodies involved in extravascular DHTRs rarely fix complement, the clinical signs and symptoms are usually much less severe than are those associated with acute intravascular HTRs. IgG-mediated phagocytosis results in inflammatory cytokine production but at a lower level than in AHTRs.[7] Because of the low level of inflammatory response and lack of complement activation, patients with DHTRs often manifest only slight fever, weakness, and symptoms referable to anemia. A positive DAT result will be caused by the coating of the transfused donor red cells with recipient antibody. Destruction of the transfused red cells may cause anemia and indirect hyperbilirubinemia. Other laboratory findings may include an elevated reticulocyte count, increased LDH, and decreased haptoglobin. Hemoglobinemia is unusual. In the rare situations when transfusion is necessary but compatible blood is not obtainable, high-dose IVIG given before transfusion may prevent a DHTR.[50]

Intravascular DHTRs also occur and often are associated with antibodies to the Duffy (Fy^a, Fy^b) or Kidd (Jk^a or Jk^b) blood group system antigens. The C5b-9 component of complement may be fixed to the red cell membrane, and hemolysis with hemoglobinemia and hemoglobinuria may occur. However, the rate of generation of C3a, C5a, proinflammatory cytokines, and other biologic response modifiers is lower than in an acute intravascular HTR; thus, the clinical symptoms in a DHTR are rarely life-threatening. If a patient shows signs of a severe transfusion reaction, however, treatment should follow that described for an acute intravascular HTR. DHTRs are also observed in ABO- and Rh-mismatched hematopoietic cell and solid organ transplants.

Posttransfusion Purpura

Posttransfusion purpura (PTP) is characterized by the onset of profound thrombocytopenia 1 to 3 weeks after transfusion. All types of blood components have been implicated in PTP. In these reactions, there is an antibody response to a platelet antigen. Most cases have been associated with antibodies to HPA-1a antigen on the glycoprotein IIb/IIIa complex, but other platelet antigens have also been implicated. The diagnosis is established by the finding of a platelet-specific antibody in an antigen-negative patient. The thrombocytopenia of PTP typically persists for 2 to 3 weeks and resolves spontaneously without treatment. The most likely pathophysiologic explanation for PTP is that, early in the course of an alloimmune response, the patient produces low-affinity antibodies that crossreact with autologous platelets. As the immune response naturally matures, low-affinity crossreacting clones are eliminated and a pure alloantibody remains. The treatment of PTP is dependent on the clinical picture. Stable patients with low risk for hemorrhage may be followed closely until the platelet count returns to normal. Patients with significant bleeding or risk for hemorrhage should receive treatment to shorten the course of thrombocytopenia. High-dose IVIG has been reported to increase the platelet count abruptly.[51] Alternatively, plasma exchange has been tried to remove the causative antibody (see Chapter 7: Therapeutic Apheresis).[52] Platelet transfusion is indicated for severe bleeding, but prophylactic platelet transfusion is futile and may delay recovery. There is no utility in transfusing antigen-negative platelets, even when a specificity is identified, because that patient is destroying perfectly matched platelets—his or her own. Steroids have not been shown to shorten the course of PTP.

Graft-vs-Host Disease

Graft-vs-host disease (GVHD), a well-recognized complication of allogeneic hematopoietic cell transplantation, can also occur after the transfusion of immunologically competent donor lymphocytes, usually to an immunoincompetent recipient.[53,54] Transfusion-associated GVHD (TA-GVHD) also has been observed after the transfusion of cellular components from HLA-homozygous donors to immunocompetent recipients who are heterozygous for the HLA haplotype.[55] Whereas the latter occurs more frequently after transfusion of blood from first- or second-degree relatives, it has been reported to occur with the transfusion of blood from unrelated HLA-homozygous donors.[56] GVHD is initiated by alloreactive donor T-cell recognition of host histocompatibility antigens.[57] Donor lymphocytes engraft in the recipient, proliferate, and attack host tissue. TA-GVHD typically begins 10 to 12 days after transfusion and is characterized by fever, skin rash, diarrhea, hepatitis, and marrow aplasia. TA-GVHD is fatal in most cases, usually because of host marrow failure that results in overwhelming infection or bleeding. TA-GVHD can be prevented by gamma irradiation of cellular blood components, which renders donor lymphocytes incapable of proliferating.[58] To prevent TA-GVHD in susceptible patients, blood and cellular components are irradiated with at least 2500 cGy.[45] In addition, all HLA-matched components and all cellular components from blood relatives should be irradiated, regardless of patient diagnosis.

Hemosiderosis

One mL of red cells contains 1 mg of iron. Therefore, an RBC unit may contain 150 to 250 mg of iron. In persons with chronic anemia, the continued need for red cell transfusion results in the accumulation of iron, which can eventually produce organ damage, particularly in the heart, liver, and pancreatic islets. There is no physiologic mechanism for the excretion of excess iron. The parenteral iron chelator deferoxamine can prevent the complications of iron overload in patients undergoing chronic red cell transfusion therapy,[59] but has a high rate of noncompliance. Better compliance may be achieved with deferasirox. Deferasirox is a daily oral iron chelator that is approved in the United States for treatment for transfusional iron overload, for patients older than 2 years of age.[60] Red cell exchange by apheresis has also been used to limit iron accumulation in patients with sickle cell disease who require repeated transfusions. (Refer to Table 11 in Chapter 7: Therapeutic Apheresis.)

Air Embolism

Air embolism is rarely a problem with conventional transfusion techniques. Rapid infusion devices can infuse as much as 200 mL of air in 4 seconds. Air embolism may also be seen with the use of intraoperative blood recovery. The frequency of fatal air embolism after the infusion of recovered blood is 1:30,000 to 1:38,000.[61] Air embolism produces acute cardiopulmonary insufficiency, because the air tends to migrate to the right ventricle, where it produces outlet obstruction. Acute cyanosis, pain, cough, arrythmia, shock, and cardiac arrest may result. Patients with a patent foramen ovale may also present with central nervous system symptoms. Immediate treatment includes placing the patient head-down on the left side in an attempt to dislodge the air bubble from the pulmonary valve.

Transfusion-Transmitted Diseases

Allogeneic blood donations are tested for the presence of hepatitis B surface antigen (HBsAg); antibody to hepatitis B core antigen (anti-HBc); antibody to hepatitis C virus (anti-HCV); antibody to human immunodeficiency virus, types 1/2 (anti-HIV-1/2); antibody to human T-cell lymphotropic virus, types I and II (anti-HTLV-I/II); a serologic test for syphilis; and nucleic acid amplification testing (NAT) for HBV, HCV, HIV, and West Nile virus (WNV). An ELISA test for antibody to *Trypanosoma cruzi* (Chagas disease) is also available but is not currently required. Despite extensive donor screening and testing, infections can still be transmitted by blood transfusion. Most transmissions of hepatitis or HIV today occur from donors in the window period between infection and the appearance of detectable antibody or virus. All cases of suspected posttransfusion infection should be reported to the blood bank, to identify infectious donors and prevent further transmissions.

Hepatitis

HCV accounts for most posttransfusion hepatitis. Almost all cases of posttransfusion HCV were acquired before the implementation of donor serologic screening in 1990. Less than 20% of acute infections are symptomatic, and 85% of infections become chronic, but they are usually asymptomatic. Among chronic carriers of HCV, cirrhosis occurs in 20% to 50% within 20 years and hepatocellular carcinoma in 15% to 20% within 30 years. In addition, chronic infection may lead to cryoglobulinemia and vasculitis.

In contrast to HCV, acute hepatitis B virus (HBV) infection is symptomatic in 30% to 50% of adults but in less than 10% of children less than 5 years old. Chronic infection occurs in 2% to 10% of adults but in 30% to 90% of children less than 5 years old. Premature death from cirrhosis or hepatocellular carcinoma occurs in 15% to 25% of chronic carriers. Recent estimates of the window period for HBV and HCV are 60 to 150 days and 16 to 32 days, respectively. Estimates of the per-unit risk of transfusion-transmitted hepatitis are 1 in 200,000 to 1 in 500,000 for HBV and approximately 1 in 2 million for HCV.[62,63] Testing for HBV by NAT found a positivity rate of 1 in 410,540 donations.[64] Hepatitis A transmission has occurred with plasma derivatives but is not a substantial risk for blood components. Hepatitis G virus may be transmitted by transfusion but does not appear to be associated with disease.

HIV

Transfusion-transmitted HIV has declined markedly since the implementation of antibody testing in 1985. The clinical manifestations of transfusion-transmitted HIV infection are similar to those of infections acquired through other routes. The current rate of transmission by transfusion is very rare. The current estimated window period for HIV is 12 to 13 days. The per-unit risk of HIV transmission is estimated to be approximately 1 in 2 million in the United States.[63]

West Nile Virus

WNV, a mosquito-borne virus primarily infecting birds, has humans as incidental hosts and thus has become a major public health concern in North America. Since 1999, WNV has caused several thousand cases of febrile illness and neuroinvasive disease such as encephalitis, meningitis, and spastic paralysis. WNV infections occur during the spring and summer months when mosquitoes are active. Evidence of transmission through transfusion, breast-feeding, and organ transplantation has been reported.[65,66] WNV NAT has been performed throughout the United States since 2003, and it has prevented many cases of potential transmission. However, the low levels of viremia in infected blood donors, especially during the early stages of infection, have required complex seasonal and temporal testing algorithms using pooled and individual donor samples.

Other Viruses

Cytomegalovirus (CMV) infection is a major concern in immunosuppressed recipients. Latent CMV infection is common among blood donors. CMV DNA can be found in the leukocytes of seropositive and seronegative donors.[67] Transmission of CMV can be significantly reduced with equivalent efficacy by the use of either seronegative or leukocyte-reduced blood components, although this continues to be debated.[68,69]

HTLVs are retroviruses unrelated to HIV. They are causally associated with adult T-cell lymphoma-leukemia and peripheral neuropathy (HTLV-associated myelopathy). HTLV-I/II infections are rare in the United States. Because these viruses are strongly associated with white cells, leukocyte reduction may further reduce their transmission by transfusion.

Parvovirus B19 causes erythema infectiosum in childhood. This virus can infect red cell precursors in marrow and, in patients with accelerated hematopoiesis, it can cause hypoplastic or aplastic anemia. Parvovirus can cause aplastic crisis in sickle cell disease, nonimmune hydrops if acquired in pregnancy, and marrow transplant failure. Parvovirus B19 is common in the general population. High-titer antibody can be found in donor plasma.[70] Transmission by blood transfusion occurs but seldom causes significant disease.[71]

Epstein-Barr virus and human herpesvirus 8 are transmissible by transfusion, but they do not appear to be of clinical significance in transfusion recipients.

The retrovirus xenotropic murine leukemia virus-related virus (XMRV) has been isolated from two-thirds of 101 patients with chronic fatigue syndrome diagnosed by a physician, and in 3.7% of 218 healthy controls. This as well as other viral characteristics has raised concerns about transfusion transmissibility of XMRV. Consequently, the AABB has advised blood collection agencies to defer potential donors diagnosed with chronic fatigue syndrome from blood donation.[72]

Parasites

Transfusion-transmitted malaria is uncommon in the United States, but it does occur.[73] The most frequently implicated species is *Plasmodium falciparum.* The mortality rate for transfusion-transmitted malaria is 10%. Exclusion of high-risk donors is the most effective preventive measure currently available. Transfusion-transmitted babesiosis has occurred in the United States, resulting in a number of deaths in the last 6 years. The parasitic reservoir is widely distributed in North America. Current serologic tests are inadequate for blood donor screening. Transfusion transmission of *T. cruzi*, the cause of Chagas disease, is a problem in areas of the world where the causative agent is endemic, and it has occurred in the United States. Serologic screening for *T. cruzi* infection may be effective when there is a high proportion of donors who emigrated from such areas. A serologic test has been licensed for the screening of blood donors in the United States, but is not required by the FDA.

Prions

Creutzfeldt-Jakob disease (CJD) is an illness caused by proteinaceous particles known as prions. Variant CJD (vCJD) differs from classical CJD in the absence of affected family members, younger age of onset, more rapid progression, and association with consumption of certain animal products. Experimental models and theoretical considerations suggest that transmission by blood components is probable.[74,75] There have been several reports of probable vCJD transmission by blood transfusion.[76,77] B cells and dendritic cells have been suggested to play a crucial role in the development of spongiform encephalopathy, and that possibility has led to the adoption of leukocyte reduction to minimize the risk of transfusion-transmitted vCJD.[78,79] However, no data exist to support universal leukocyte reduction as an efficacious method in preventing the spread of vCJD by transfused blood. At present, there is no practical donor screening test for the abnormal isoform of the prion protein, although progress in test development is being made.[80] Current strategies for reducing the theoretical risk of prion transmission include deferral of donors with a family history of CJD, exposure to risk factors, or residence or blood transfusion in vCJD-endemic regions.

Hemovigilance

In 2006, the US Department of Health and Human Services and the private-sector blood collection, transfusion, tissue and organ transplant organizations initiated a collaboration to monitor adverse events associated with transfusion and transplantation. The hemovigilance module of the Centers for Disease Control and Prevention's National Healthcare Safety Network,[81] the first system developed under this collaboration, began to track adverse events of transfusion in February, 2010 with a goal of improvement to patient safety.

References

1. Food and Drug Administration. Fatalities reported to FDA following blood collection and transfusion: Annual summary for fiscal year (FY) 2009. Rockville, MD: CBER Office of Communication, Outreach, and Development. [Available at http://www.fda.gov/BiologicsBloodVaccines/SafetyAvailability/ReportaProblem/TransfusionDonationFatalities/ucm204763.htm.]

2. Davenport RD. Hemolytic transfusion reactions. In: Popovsky MA, ed. Transfusion reactions. 3rd ed. Bethesda, MD: AABB Press, 2007:1-55.

3. Petz L, Garratty G. The diagnosis of hemolytic anemia. In: Immune hemolytic anemias. 2nd ed. Philadelphia: Churchill Livingstone, 2004:48-9.

4. Gladwin MT. Role of the red blood cell in nitric oxide homeostasis and hypoxic vasodilation. Adv Exp Med Biol 2006;588:189-205.

5. Davenport RD. Inflammatory cytokines in hemolytic transfusion reactions. In: Davenport RD, Snyder EL, eds. Cytokines in transfusion medicine: A primer. Bethesda, MD: AABB Press, 1997:85-97.

6. Butler J, Parker D, Pillai R, et al. Systemic release of neutrophil elastase and tumour necrosis factor alpha following ABO incompatible blood transfusion. Br J Haematol 1991;79:525-6.

7. Davenport RD, Burdick M, Moore SA, Kunkel SL. Cytokine production in IgG-mediated red cell incompatibility. Transfusion 1993;33:19-24.

8. Pierce RN, Reich LM, Mayer K. Hemolysis following platelet transfusions from ABO-incompatible donors. Transfusion 1985;25:60-2.

9. Kim HC, Park CL, Cowan JH, et al. Massive intravascular hemolysis associated with intravenous immunoglobulin in

bone marrow transplant recipients. Am J Pediatr Hematol Oncol 1988;10:69-74.

10. Mair B, Benson K. Evaluation of changes in hemoglobin levels associated with ABO-incompatible plasma in apheresis platelets. Transfusion 1998;38:51-5.

11. Petz LD, Calhoun L, Shulman IA, et al. The sickle cell hemolytic transfusion reaction syndrome. Transfusion 1997;37:382-92.

12. King KE, Shirey RS, Lankiewicz MW, et al. Delayed hemolytic transfusion reactions in sickle cell disease: Simultaneous destruction of recipients' red cells. Transfusion 1997;37:376-81.

13. Telen MJ, Combs M. Management of massive delayed hemolytic transfusion reactions in patients with sickle cell disease (abstract). Transfusion 1999;39(Suppl):443S.

14. Win N, Sinha S, Lee E, Mills W. Treatment with intravenous immunoglobulin and steroids may correct severe anemia in hyperhemolytic transfusion reactions: Case report and literature review. Transfus Med Rev 2010;24:64-7.

15. Chadebech P, Habibi AN, Nzouakou R, et al. Delayed hemolytic transfusion reaction in sickle cell disease patients: Evidence of an emerging syndrome with suicidal red blood cell death. Transfusion 2009;49:1785-92.

16. Johnson ST, Fueger JT, Gottschall JL. One center's experience: The serology and drugs associated with drug-induced hemolytic anemia—a new paradigm. Transfusion 2007; 47:697-702.

17. Perkins HA, Payne R, Ferguson J, Wood M. Nonhemolytic febrile transfusion reactions. Quantitative effects of blood components with emphasis on isoantigenic incompatibility of leukocytes. Vox Sang 1966;11:578-99.

18. Heddle NM, Kelton JG. Febrile nonhemolytic transfusion reactions. In: Popovsky MA, ed. Transfusion reactions. 3rd ed. Bethesda, MD: AABB Press, 2007:45-82.

19. Mangano MM, Chambers LA, Kruskall MS. Limited efficacy of leukopoor platelets for prevention of febrile transfusion reactions. Am J Clin Pathol 1991;95:733-8.

20. Lane TA, Anderson KC, Goodnough LT, et al. Leukocyte reduction in blood component therapy. Ann Intern Med 1992;117:151-62.

21. Aye MT, Palmer DS, Giulivi A, et al. Effects of filtration of platelet concentrates on the accumulation of cytokines and platelet release factors during storage. Transfusion 1995; 35:117-24.

22. King KE, Shirey RS, Thoman SK, et al. Universal leukoreduction decreases the incidence of febrile nonhemolytic transfusion reactions to RBCs. Transfusion 2004;44:25-9.

23. Phipps RP, Kaufman J, Blumberg N. Platelet derived CD154 (CD40 ligand) and febrile responses to transfusion. Lancet 2001;357:2023-4.

24. Geiger TL, Howard SC. Acetaminophen and diphenhydramine premedication for allergic and febrile nonhemolytic transfusion reactions: Good prophylaxis or bad practice? Transfus Med Rev 2007;21:1-12.

25. Domen RE, Hoeltge GA. Allergic transfusion reactions: An evaluation of 273 consecutive reactions. Arch Pathol Lab Med 2003;127:316-20.

26. Vyas GN, Perkins HA, Fudenberg HH. Anaphylactoid transfusion reactions associated with anti-IgA. Lancet 1968;ii:12-15.

27. Westhoff CM, Sipherd BD, Wylie DE, Toalson LD. Severe anaphylactic reaction following transfusion of platelets to a patient with anti-Ch. Transfusion 1992;32:576-9.

28. Koda Y, Watanabe Y, Soejima M, et al. Simple PCR detection of haptoglobin gene deletion in anhaptoglobinemic patients with antihaptoglobin antibody that causes anaphylactic transfusion reactions. Blood 2000;95:1138-43.

29. Davenport RD, Burnie KL, Barr RM. Transfusion management of patients with IgA deficiency and anti-IgA during liver transplantation. Vox Sang 1992;63:247-50.

30. Kennedy L, Case L, Hurd D, et al. A prospective, randomized, double-blind controlled trial of acetaminophen and diphenhydramine pretransfusion medication versus pla-

cebo for the prevention of transfusion reactions. Transfusion 2008;48:2285-91.

31. Popovsky MA. Transfusion and lung injury. Transfus Clin Biol 2001;8:272-7.

32. Kleinman S, Caulfield T, Chan P, et al. Toward an understanding of transfusion-related lung injury: Statement of a consensus panel. Transfusion 2004;44:1774-89.

33. Silliman CC, Ambrusco DR, Boshkov LK. Transfusion-related acute lung injury (TRALI). Blood 2005;105:2266-73.

34. Popovsky MA, Davenport RD. Transfusion-related acute lung injury: Femme fatale? Transfusion 2001;41:312-5.

35. Silliman CC, Paterson AJ, Dickey WO, et al. The association of biologically active lipids with the development of transfusion-related acute lung injury: A retrospective study. Transfusion 1997;37:719-26.

36. Toy P, Hollis-Perry KM, Jun J, et al. Recipients of blood from a donor with multiple HLA antibodies: A lookback study of transfusion-related acute lung injury. Transfusion 2004;44:1683-8.

37. Kopko PM, Marshall CS, MacKenzie MR, et al. Transfusion-related acute lung injury: Report of a clinical lookback investigation. JAMA 2002;287:1968-71.

38. Clarifications to recommendations to reduce the risk of TRALI. Association bulletin 07-03. Bethesda, MD: AABB, 2007.

39. Shiba M, Tadokoro K, Sawanobori M, et al. Activation of the contact system by filtration of platelet concentrates with a negatively charged white cell-removal filter and measurement of venous blood bradykinin level in patients who received filtered platelets. Transfusion 1997;37:457-62.

40. Hild M, Soderstrom T, Egberg N, et al. Kinetics of bradykinin levels during and after leucocyte filtration of platelet concentrates. Vox Sang 1998;75:18-25.

41. Mair B, Leparc GF. Hypotensive reactions associated with platelet transfusions and angiotensin-converting enzyme inhibitors. Vox Sang 1998;74:27-30.

42. De Korte D, Marcelis JH, Soeterboek AM. Determination of the degree of bacterial contamination of whole-blood collections using an automated microbe-detection system. Transfusion 2001;41:815-8.
43. Perez P, Salmi LR, Folléa G, et al. Determinants of transfusion-associated bacterial contamination: Results of the French BACTHEM Case-Control Study. Transfusion 2001;41:862-72.
44. Guidance on implementation of new bacteria reduction and detection standard (supersedes association bulletin #03-07). Association bulletin #03-10. Bethesda, MD: AABB, 2003.
45. Eder A, Kennedy J, Dy B, et al. Bacterial screening of apheresis platelets and the residual risk of septic transfusion reactions: The American Red Cross experience (2004-2006). Transfusion 2007;47:1134-42.
46. Dzik WH, Kirkley SA. Citrate toxicity during massive blood transfusion. Transfus Med Rev 1988;2:76-94.
47. Weiskopf R, Schnapp S, Rouine-Rapp K, et al. Extracellular potassium concentrations in red blood cell suspensions after irradiation and washing. Transfusion 2005;45:1295-301.
48. Driscoll DF, Bistrian BR, Jenkins RL, et al. Development of metabolic alkalosis after massive transfusion during orthotopic liver transplantation. Crit Care Med 1987;15:905-8.
49. Zimring JC. Principles of red blood cell alloimmunization and autoantibody formation and function. In: Hillyer CD, Silberstein, L, Ness, PM, et al, eds. Blood banking and transfusion medicine: Basic principles and practice. 2nd ed. Philadelphia: Churchill Livingstone, 2007:43-52.
50. Kohan AI, Niborski RC, Rey JA, et al. High-dose intravenous immunoglobulin in non-ABO transfusion incompatibility. Vox Sang 1994;67:195-8.
51. Mueller-Eckhardt C. Post-transfusion purpura. Br J Haematol 1986;64:419-24.

52. Laursen B, Morling N, Rosenkvist J, et al. Post-transfusion purpura treated with plasma exchange by Haemonetics cell separator. Acta Med Scand 1978;203:539-43.
53. Linden JV, Pisciotto PT. Transfusion-associated graft-versus-host disease and blood irradiation. Transfus Med Rev 1992;6:116-23.
54. Holland PV. Prevention of transfusion-associated graft-vs-host disease. Arch Pathol Lab Med 1989;113:285-91.
55. Thaler M, Shamiss A, Orgad S, et al. The role of blood from HLA homozygous donors in fatal transfusion-associated graft-versus-host disease after open heart surgery. N Engl J Med 1989;321:25-8.
56. Shivdasani RA, Haluska FG, Dock NL, et al. Graft-versus-host disease associated with transfusion of blood from unrelated HLA-homozygous donors. N Engl J Med 1993; 328:766-70.
57. Krenger W, Ferrara JLM. Dysregulation of cytokines during graft-versus-host disease. J Hematother 1996;5:3-14.
58. Moroff G, Luban NLC. The irradiation of blood and blood components to prevent graft-versus-host disease: Technical issues and guidelines. Transfus Med Rev 1997;11:15-26.
59. Marcus CS, Huehns ER. Transfusional iron overload. Clin Lab Haematol 1985;7:195-212.
60. Delea T, Edelsberg J, Sofrygin O, et al. Consequences and costs of noncompliance with iron chelation treatment in patients with transfusion dependent thalassemia: A literature review. Transfusion 2007;47:1919-29.
61. Linden J, Kaplan H, Murphy MT. Fatal air embolism due to perioperative blood recovery. Anesth Analg 1997;84: 422-6.
62. Stramer SL. Current risks of transfusion-transmitted agents: A review. Arch Pathol Lab Med 2007;131:702-7.
63. Stramer SL, Glynn SA, Kleinman SH, et al. Detection of HIV-1 and HCV infections among antibody-negative blood donors by nucleic-acid amplification testing. N Engl J Med 2004;351:760-8.

64. Stramer S, Wend U, Candotti D, et al. Nucleic acid testing to detect HBV infection in blood donors. N Engl J Med 2011;364:236-47.

65. Iwamoto M, Jernigan DB, Guasch A, et al. Transmission of West Nile virus from an organ donor to four transplant recipients. N Engl J Med 2003;348:2196-203.

66. Pealer LN, Marfin AA, Lanciotti RS, et al. Transmission of West Nile virus through blood transfusion in the United States, 2002. N Engl J Med 2003;349:1236-45.

67. Larsson S, Soderberg-Naucler C, Wang FZ, Moller E. Cytomegalovirus DNA can be detected in peripheral blood mononuclear cells from all seropositive and most seronegative healthy blood donors over time. Transfusion 1998;38:271-8.

68. Bowden RA, Slichter SJ, Sayers M, et al. A comparison of filtered leukocyte-reduced and cytomegalovirus (CMV) seronegative blood products for the prevention of transfusion-associated CMV infection after marrow transplantation. Blood 1995;86:3598-603.

69. Nichols WB, Price TH, Gooley T, et al. Transfusion-transmitted cytomegalovirus infection after receipt of leukoreduced blood. Blood 2003;101:4195-200.

70. Weimer T, Streichert S, Watson C, Gršner A. High-titer screening PCR: A successful strategy for reducing the parvovirus B19 load in plasma pools for fractionation. Transfusion 2001;41:1500-4.

71. Koenigbauer UF, Eastland T, Day JW. Clinical illness due to parvovirus B19 infection after infusion of solvent/detergent-treated pooled plasma. Transfusion 2000;40:1203-6.

72. Klein HG, Dodd RY, Hollinger FB, et al. Xenotropic murine leukemia virus-related virus (XMRV) and blood transfusion: Report of the AABB interorganizational XMRV task force. Transfusion 2011;51:643-53.

73. Mungai M, Tegtmeier G, Chamberland M, Parise M. Transfusion-transmitted malaria in the United States from 1963 through 1999. N Engl J Med 2001;344:1973-8.

74. Brown P, Rohwer RG, Dunstan BC, et al. The distribution of infectivity in blood components and plasma derivatives in experimental models of transmissible spongiform encephalopathy. Transfusion 1998;38:810-6.

75. Houston F, Foster JD, Chong A, et al. Transmission of BSE by blood transfusion in sheep. Lancet 2000;356:999-1000.

76. Llewelyn CA, Hewitt PE, Knight RSG, et al. Possible transmission of variant Creutzfeldt-Jakob disease by blood transfusion. Lancet 2004;364:527-9.

77. Peden AH, Head MW, Ritchie DL, et al. Preclinical vCJD after blood transfusion in a PRNP codon 129 heterozygous patient. Lancet 2004;364:527-9.

78. Klein MA, Frigg R, Flechsig E, et al. A crucial role for B cells in neuroinvasive scrapie. Nature 1997;390:687-90.

79. Klein MA, Frigg R, Raeber AJ, et al. PrP expression in B lymphocytes is not required for prion neuroinvasion. Nat Med 1998;4:1429-33.

80. MacGregor I. Prion protein and developments in its detection. Transfus Med 2001;11:3-14.

81. US Biovigilance Network. Investing in patient safety and donor health. Bethesda, MD: AABB, 2010. [Available at http://www.aabb.org/programs/biovigilance/us/Pages/default.aspx (accessed May 13, 2011).]

HEMATOPOIETIC CELLULAR THERAPY

Concept of Hematopoietic Therapy

Hematopoietic progenitor cells (HPCs) are primitive cells with capabilities of self-renewal and differentiation into committed hematopoietic cells. Recently, HPCs were also shown to dedifferentiate and transdifferentiate into nonhematopoietic cells.[1] HPCs are best categorized by their ability to form colony-forming units (CFUs) and long-term culture-initiating cells. These stem cells express CD34+ antigens and lack the expression of hematopoietic lineage-committed antigens. Sources of hematopoietic stem cells include marrow, peripheral blood, and cord blood. The choices for stem cell sources are influenced by the availability, best-matched donor, and safety and complications of the donor. HPCs may be obtained from the patient (autologous), from an identical twin (syngeneic), or from a related or unrelated individual (allogeneic). Allogeneic HPCs are used therapeutically for the treatment of hematologic malignancies, marrow failure, immunodeficiency syndromes, some hemoglobinopathies, and inborn errors of metabolism. Autologous HPC therapy is used in the treatment of hematologic and other malignancies and nonmalignant conditions (ie, autoimmune disorders).

HPC donor selection falls under the regulatory oversight of the Food and Drug Administration (FDA) for peripheral-blood-derived stem cell sources and the Health Resources and Services Administration (HRSA) for marrow-derived stem cell sources. Donor selection regulations require screening for infectious diseases by history and laboratory testing. The primary infectious diseases that donors are screened for include human immunodeficiency virus (HIV), hepatitis C virus, hepatitis B virus, human T-cell lymphotropic virus (HTLV), and syphilis. Individuals are declared to be either an "eligible donor" or an "ineligible donor" based on the donor screening process.

In autologous transplantation, HPCs are primarily used for hematopoietic "rescue" in patients who have received myeloablative therapy (ie, chemotherapy and/or radiation). In allogeneic HPC transplantation, there is an additional benefit: T cells in the graft attack residual tumor cells in what has been called the graft-vs-leukemia effect. These T cells also mediate the primary complication of allogeneic HPC therapy, graft-vs-host disease (GVHD), which results in the higher transplant-related morbidity and mortality than is seen with autologous HPC therapy. Furthermore, emerging data suggest that relapse of acute leukemia following allogeneic HPC transplantation may be related to the donor cells in as high as 5% of patients.[2] HPCs are also used to reconstitute marrow function in marrow failure syndromes such as aplastic anemia or to restore immune function in immunodeficiency states.

In the near future, HPCs could serve as a vehicle for gene therapy, such as in the treatment of severe combined immunodeficiency. Breakthrough discoveries about the plasticity of adult stem cells showed that HPCs potentially can be used to generate a variety of nonhematopoietic tissue cell types, such as heart, lung, liver, muscle, and brain.[3,4] Advances in the collection and processing of HPCs, development of the capability to expand hematopoietic cells, and the promise of solid organ repair and gene therapy are likely to increase the study of and indications for HPC therapy.

Marrow-Derived HPCs

Description of Component

HPCs derived from marrow (HPC, Marrow) may be obtained from autologous, syngeneic, or allogeneic donors. Collections are harvested from hematopoietically active, readily accessible skeletal sites, usually the iliac crests in adults. Harvesting is performed in the operating room under general, spinal, or epidural anesthesia, and it is accomplished by multiple punctures and aspirations of the iliac crest. Marrow is aspirated into citrate or heparin anticoagulant and filtered (200- to 500-micron pore size) to remove clots, bone fragments, and fat. About 0.5 to 1.5 L of marrow (10-15 mL/kg donor weight) is harvested from adults and contains approximately 1.0 to 1.5×10^{10} nucleated cells, exclusive of nucleated red cells.[5] It is variably diluted with peripheral blood, depending on the harvesting procedure. Autologous marrow may also contain malignant cells if they are present in the patient's marrow. Marrow may be processed in the laboratory 1) to prevent hemolysis by removing donor plasma antibodies that are incompatible with recipient red cells or by removing donor red cells that are incompatible with recipient plasma antibodies; 2) to diminish or eliminate autologous malignant cells that might contribute to disease relapse; 3) to diminish the severity of GVHD by reducing the content of donor T cells; or 4) to accomplish all of the above and reduce overall volume by the selection and concentration of early HPCs (eg, cells that carry the CD34 antigen).[6] Consequently, the final product may have a variable volume, hematocrit, and cell concentration. HPC, Marrow may be stored frozen in a cryopreservative that contains dimethylsulfoxide (DMSO). The cryopreserved product must be transfused as soon as possible after thawing to maintain cell viability. Fresh noncryopreserved products can be stored at refrigerated temperatures (ie, 4 C) for up to 72 hrs before transfusion and retain cell viability.[7] Once donor HPC, Marrow cells are transplanted, neutrophils engraft in about 3 weeks, which is approximately 1 week longer compared to HPC, Apheresis grafts.[8]

Indications

Allogeneic and syngeneic collections are intended to provide permanent lymphohematopoietic engraftment after transplantation. Marrow may be indicated in certain settings because of the donor's preference for a harvesting method or because of the donor's prior failure to mobilize peripheral blood progenitor cells.

Potential allogeneic marrow donors must be HLA-matched with the recipient to ensure engraftment and diminish the risk of GVHD. Donor and recipient blood types must also be identified to assess compatibility and to determine the need for additional marrow processing. This may involve either the removal of incompatible red cells from the marrow for major ABO-incompatible transplants or the removal of plasma from the marrow for minor ABO-incompatible transplants.[9] This processing is performed to prevent hemolysis of donor or recipient red cells.

Contraindications and Precautions

The National Marrow Donor Program (NMDP) is a federally supported organization dedicated to forwarding safe and effective HPC transplantation worldwide. Regarding matched unrelated donor safety, the NMDP works closely with teams to monitor the volume of marrow collected, the type and duration of the anesthesia, and the incidence of acute and chronic donor complications. The NMDP has reported that serious medical complications occur in 1.3% of marrow donors. These complications include infections, mechanical injuries, and reactions to anesthesia. The incidence of minor complications was 82%, and included back pain, throat pain, and postanesthesia headache.[10] In addition, many donors were anemic after collection. NMDP standards require marrow volume not to exceed 20 mL/kg of donor body weight, because a larger volume may lead a donor to require a transfusion.[10,11] Nevertheless, volume loss is expected during donation and the harvested marrow volume is usually repleted using banked autologous blood and crystalloid. Approximately 80% to 90% of healthy donors will receive autologous banked blood.[10,12]

Allogeneic marrow transplantation carries a relatively high risk of recipient mortality and is performed only in facilities with a specially trained transplant team. Recipient risks inherent in marrow transplantation include those associated with treatment (conditioning), regimen toxicity (eg, veno-occlusive disease of the liver or interstitial pulmonary disease), prolonged cytopenia (eg, infections or hemorrhage), immune suppression [eg, reactivation of cytomegalovirus (CMV) infection], and disease relapse. Risks associated with the graft include an inadequate HPC dose, failure to engraft, rejection of the graft, GVHD, hemolysis caused by donor-recipient red cell incompatibility, infection caused by microbial contamination, transmission of viral infection, and acute reactions associated with the infusion of lysed granulocytes or DMSO.[13]

Common side effects of DMSO include an unpleasant taste in the mouth and a "garlic or metallic" smell on the breath, nausea, vomiting, diarrhea, chills, and hypertension. Anaphylactoid reactions (eg, flushing, hypotension, bronchospasm, and pulmonary edema) may also occur because of the release of bradykinin and histamine. Cardiovascular effects such as cardiac arrhythmias and neurologic symptoms are multifactorial and commonly observed. DMSO toxicity, hypervolemia, and hypothermia contribute to symptoms such as bradycardia and/or headache. More symptoms occur when HPC, Apheresis cells are infused as compared to HPC, Marrow cells; however, HPC, Marrow infusions are associated with more severe bradycardic events.[14]

Dose and Administration

The minimal effective dose has not been clearly established, but the usual minimum recommended dose is 2×10^8 nucleated cells/kg recipient body weight.[15] However, centers are increasingly using the measurement of CD34+ cells (or CD34+ subsets) to assess cell dose. Studies suggest that a CD34+ dose less than 1 $\times 10^6$ CD34+ cells/kg is associated with a higher transplant-related mortality and a dose greater than 2×10^6 CD34+ cells/kg is associated with earlier mononuclear cell recovery.[16] It is common practice to administer marrow with or without a standard blood filter. However, a leukocyte reduction filter must *never* be used during marrow transfusion, because leukocyte reduction filters remove hematopoietic cells. Likewise, HPC, Marrow should *never* be irradiated, because irradiation will prevent HPCs from engrafting.[17] The optimal storage temperature and the upper limit of shelf life have not been defined, but it has been recommended that marrow should be transfused as soon as practical after processing, preferably within 24 hours.[11] Marrow shipped overnight at room temperature has successfully engrafted in patients treated through the NMDP. The cryopreserved product is generally thawed at the bedside between 37 and 40 C and transfused immediately without filtration, preferably through a central venous catheter. Unlike blood components, marrow for transplantation represents an irreplaceable life-sparing biologic product that is specifically designated for a given patient. Consequently, extra effort must be made to ensure that the product is properly handled, that cell viability is maintained during storage and transport, and that the recipient receives the product in a timely manner.

HPCs Obtained by Apheresis

Description of Component

Very small numbers of HPCs are found in the peripheral blood of healthy individuals. The number of circulating HPCs may be increased (or "mobilized" from the marrow) up to 100-fold or higher by administration of hematopoietic growth factors such as granulocyte colony-stimulating factor (G-CSF) and granulocyte-macrophage colony-stimulating factor (GM-CSF) (see Hematopoietic Growth Factors below). These mobilized stem cells can be collected from the peripheral blood using apheresis (HPC, Apheresis) technology.

Both healthy donors and patients can have their stem cells harvested with apheresis equipment. However, whereas healthy donors have their stem cells mobilized using growth factor alone, patients often receive growth factors in conjunction with the rebound of the leukocyte count from chemotherapy-induced cytopenia. Growth factor plus chemotherapy to mobilize stem cells is used for autologous transplantation.[18-21] Mobilized HPCs are collected by one or more leukapheresis procedures during which two or more blood volumes (10-24 L) are processed, typically yielding 1 to 8×10^{10} leukocytes containing 0.1% to 5% CD34+ leukocytes. Some centers perform a single large-volume apheresis collection with good results.[22] The quality of apheresis collection is based on the number of cells bearing the CD34 antigen. Usually only 1% to 2% of the mononuclear cells (MNCs) in the apheresis collection express the CD34 antigen. However, a greater number of CD34+ cells can be collected by increasing either the number of cells mobilized or the number of procedures and/or volume of blood processed.[23,24] Apheresis products may be stored frozen in a cryopreservative containing DMSO. After thawing, the product must be transfused as soon as possible to maintain viability.

Indications

HPC, Apheresis may be used alone or, more rarely, as a supplement to HPC, Marrow transfusion for autologous or allogeneic transplantation. Potential advantages in the use of mobilized apheresis preparations include a diminished duration of severe cytopenia after transplant (8-10 days for neutrophil engraftment and 10-12 days for platelet engraftment), avoidance of donor hospitalization, avoidance of general anesthesia during collection, and reduced incidence of tumor cell contamination in autologous transplantation.[25] Challenges with apheresis collections

187

include some difficulty in determining the optimal timing of leukapheresis, vascular access problems, and the need to perform multiple leukapheresis procedures to collect sufficient numbers of progenitor cells, especially in poorly mobilized patients. Generally, apheresis collection can start with a peripheral blood CD34+ count as low as 5 cells/μL, but, if possible, it should start with a CD34+ count of at least 10 to 20 cells/μL. Studies show that sufficient numbers of progenitor cells to perform syngeneic and allogeneic transplants can be mobilized into the peripheral blood of normal donors with use of G-CSF or the pegylated or glycosylated analogs.[24,26]

Contraindications and Precautions

Administration of hematopoietic growth factors and apheresis collection exposes the donor to different risks than does marrow harvest. In general, apheresis donors experience G-CSF-related adverse events, and marrow donors experience harvest-related adverse events.[27] To date, there are few convincing data to support the possibility that G-CSF may promote hematologic malignancies in the donor.[28] However, other risks are associated with collections such as G-CSF-associated thrombocytopenia. An apheresis donor's platelet count further decreases 20% to 30% with each HPC collection and may remain reduced from 4 to 6 days after the last collection. Depending on the degree of platelet decrease, G-CSF-associated thrombocytopenia may place a donor at risk for hemorrhage. In addition, growth factor administration is infrequently associated with thrombosis, cutaneous vasculitis, iritis, splenic rupture, and acute gouty arthritis.[29] The transfusion of multiple collections from poorly mobilized donors often results in an increased incidence and severity of infusion toxicity because of the large number of granulocytes, DMSO exposure, and volume infused. Because DMSO toxicity is dose-dependent, it is recommended that a safe maximum human intravenous (IV) dose of DMSO is 1 mL/kg/day.[6]

Dose and Administration

Most centers target a dose of >2 to 6 × 10⁶ CD34+ cells/kg of recipient body weight to ensure rapid hematopoietic engraftment.[24] The exact minimum dose is uncertain, and transplants at a dose of 2 to 3 × 10⁶ CD34+ cells/kg recipient body weight have been shown to be effective. However, if T cells are removed from the concentrate to reduce the incidence of chronic GVHD, then higher doses of CD34+ cells should be collected, because possibly half of the concentrate will be lost during cellular depletion processing.[23]

Apheresis collections can be safely frozen in 10% DMSO by either a controlled- or uncontrolled-rate freezing process.[30] Once frozen, the HPC product is typically stored in vapor phase of liquid nitrogen, but some laboratories may still maintain some liquid-phase storage freezers. Products can also be frozen in a mechanical freezer at <–80 C. The optimal storage temperature and upper limit of shelf life have not been defined. The frozen product should be infused as soon as practical after thawing or as soon as possible after processing. The use of leukocyte reduction filters and irradiation is contraindicated.

HPCs from Cord Blood

Cord blood obtained from a delivered placenta is known to be rich in early and committed progenitor cells. Since the first cord blood transplant was reported in 1989 for Fanconi anemia, more than 2000 patients have been given HPCs from cord blood (HPC, Cord Blood) for a variety of malignant and nonmalignant conditions.[31-33] The great majority of cord blood transplants are from unrelated donors, and approximately 10% to 15% are from sibling donors.[34] Cord blood is collected from the placenta at the time of delivery by using either an open or closed system. The volume is typically 80 to 100 mL (range 40-240 mL) with a mean total nucleated cell (TNC) content of $1.4 \times 10^9 \pm 1.0 \times$

10^9.[35] The CD34 cell content has been reported to be $1.4 \times 10^6 \pm 1.8 \times 10^6$ cells/kg (0.01% to 1.0% of nucleated cells).[36] Clinical studies have reported successful engraftment in children,[33,36] with a higher risk of delayed engraftment or graft failure in patients receiving $<3.7 \times 10^7$ TNC/kg or weighing more than 45 kg. The median time to neutrophil engraftment [absolute neutrophil count (ANC) >500/µL)] is 30 days and that to platelet engraftment (platelet count >20,000/µL) is 56 days.[33] Whereas neutrophil engraftment is similar to that observed after allogeneic HPC, Marrow transplantation, platelet engraftment appears to be delayed.[34] Time to engraftment is highly correlated with TNC ($>3.7 \times 10^7$ nucleated cells/kg) and total CD34+ cell dose ($>1.7 \times 10^5$ CD34+ cells/kg). A series of adult cord blood transplants have infused a target dose of 3×10^7 TNC/kg of patient body weight with a minimum dose of 1.1×10^7 TNC/kg. To achieve this dose, it was necessary to use more than one cord blood product in 85% of patients and 92% achieved neutrophil recovery in 12 days.[37] Although a 6/6 HLA-matched cord blood transplant is preferred, 5/6 HLA-matched cord blood transplants can be successful if the CD34 cell counts are high.[38] Clinical studies have also suggested that unrelated-donor cord blood transplants are associated with a lower risk of GVHD in children than are unrelated-donor marrow transplants.[33,36] However, acceptable rates of severe acute and chronic GVHD have been seen in adult transplant recipients with use of umbilical cord blood from unrelated donors.[37]

The advantages of cord blood transplantation include no risk to the donor, a lower risk of viral infection, the potential availability of cord blood from ethnic minorities that are underrepresented in the NMDP and other donor registries, more rapid availability of cells for transplantation, and a lower risk of GVHD. Disadvantages include ethical and consent issues that may arise from products collected from underage donors, allocation of cord blood to unrelated patients as the product is irreplaceable, ownership of the product, and linkage of information between donor and patient.[39] In addition, concerns remain about engraftment in adults as a result of the limited number of nucleated cells in the product. Techniques for ex-vivo expansion and pooling of collections are currently under investigation. Ex-vivo expansion of CD34+ umbilical cord cells using cytokines and serum-free media can produce stem cells that transdifferentiate into other lineages, such as natural killer cells.[40]

Donor Leukocyte Infusion

Donor leukocyte infusion (DLI) has been used increasingly after allogeneic transplantation.[41] DLI cells are collected from the HPC transplant donor. Indications for DLI include treatment of relapsed chronic myelogenous leukemia and, less frequently, acute myelogenous leukemia or acute lymphocytic leukemia. In one study, DLI was able to stimulate a graft-vs-myeloma effect, but only 58% of the patients in the study received the DLI because of toxicities associated with the transplant.[42] The presumed mechanism for DLI is a graft-vs-leukemia effect. However, DLI is also used for treatment of posttransplant Epstein-Barr virus (EBV) or CMV infection by restoring cell-mediated immunity in the recipient. A typical DLI dose for treatment of relapsed leukemia is 1×10^7 to 1×10^8 CD3+ cells/kg of recipient body weight for related transplants and one log fewer for unrelated transplants.[43] A smaller dose, similar to unrelated DLI, is required for treatment of CMV or EBV infection.[44] Complications of DLI include GVHD and the development of severe GVHD is a contraindication to further DLI.[6]

Hematopoietic Growth Factors

Erythropoietin

Erythropoietin (EPO) is a glycoprotein growth factor that stimulates the division and differentiation of committed red cell precursors in the marrow. EPO prepared by recombinant DNA technology (rHuEPO) has been approved for use in anemic patients with chronic renal failure (serum creatinine >1.8 mg/dL) to stimulate red cell production and reduce the need for RBC transfusions.[45,46] The approved dose is 50 to 100 U/kg body weight given intravenously or subcutaneously one to three times per week. This dose is reduced when the hematocrit reaches 30% to 34%. rHuEPO has also been approved to treat anemia in patients with HIV who are taking zidovudine and have endogenous EPO levels <500 mU/mL and in cancer patients undergoing chemotherapy.[47] One study has shown that there may be a quality-of-life benefit in chemotherapy patients treated with rHuEPO.[48] rHuEPO has shown some efficacy in other investigational settings, including the anemia of chronic disease, the anemia of prematurity, marrow transplantation, and autologous blood donation.[45] It also has been shown to be beneficial in a subset of patients with myelodysplastic syndrome and aplastic anemia, but it is of questionable benefit in sickle cell disease, in surgical blood loss, and in patients in the intensive care unit.[45,49] The use of EPO in many clinical settings has been questioned because of the FDA response to the CHOIR trial. The CHOIR trial showed increased severe complications such as thrombosis and myocardial infarction in patients maintained at a higher hemoglobin (13.5 g/dL) using EPO.[50] Based on these data, the FDA has required a black box warning for erythropoietin that recommends that physicians do not maintain patient hemoglobin values above 13 g/dL for any patient population, including cancer or chronic renal failure patients.[51] In response to the FDA, professional society guidelines have been updated to assist in EPO management of cancer patients.[52] Another more rare complication of EPO administration is the potential to develop red cell aplasia caused by EPO antibodies. Patients receiving rHuEPO may require iron supplementation to ensure adequate iron stores for erythropoiesis.

Novel erythropoiesis-stimulating protein or NESP (darbepoetin alfa, Aranesp, Amgen, Thousand Okas, CA), is an erythropoietin analog with a longer half-life and greater activity than EPO.

In patients with anemia and chronic renal insufficiency, once-weekly darbepoetin alfa, given intravenously or subcutaneously, has been shown to be as effective as EPO given twice weekly.[53] The FDA has approved darbepoetin alfa for the treatment of anemia caused by chronic renal failure and anemia resulting from chemotherapy. Darbepoetin alfa shares a similar black box warning as erythropoietin.

Colony-Stimulating Factors

The cloning of genes encoding the human growth factors has led to clinical trials of several myeloid colony-stimulating factors.[26,45] These factors are used alone or in combination to stimulate the proliferation and differentiation of hematopoietic progenitors. These factors appear to reduce the period of neutropenia after cytotoxic chemotherapy administration and HPC transplantation and are mainstay therapy in progenitor cell mobilization protocols.[26,54] Two of these factors have been approved for clinical use. G-CSF exerts its primary in-vivo effects on late progenitors known as granulocyte-macrophage colony-forming units (CFU-GM). G-CSF not only exerts its effects on the late CFU-GM, but it also works either directly or synergistically with other hematopoietic growth factors to stimulate progenitor cell growth.

The circulating leukocyte count rapidly increases when progenitor cells respond to exogenously administered cytokine. This leukocytosis reflects both a release of mature neutrophils from the storage pool and a decrease in the cycling time for mature progenitors. G-CSF decreases the duration of neutropenia and the incidence of infection in patients undergoing myelosuppressive chemotherapy.

G-CSF has also been used successfully in certain investigational settings, including congenital agranulocytosis, acute leukemia, myelodysplastic syndrome, aplastic anemia in children, leukopenia in AIDS, and the mobilization of HPCs for autologous or allogeneic marrow transplantation.[26,55] The combination of G-CSF and dexamethasone given the evening before granulocytapheresis (normal donors) greatly enhances the yield of collected granulocytes.[56] Like G-CSF, GM-CSF enhances the function of mature myeloid cell lines. It has been used to accelerate myeloid recovery in patients undergoing marrow transplantation and chemotherapy. Most centers use a dose of G-CSF greater than 7.5 mg/kg/day administered via a subcutaneous injection. Side effects seen with G-CSF and GM-CSF include bone pain, myalgias, anorexia, and fever. When GM-CSF is used at high doses (eg, >15 mg/kg), fluid retention, pericarditis, pleural effusions, and serositis have occurred.[57] A polyethylene glycol derivative preparation of G-CSF, pegfilgrastim (Neulasta, Amgen, Thousand Oaks, CA), is approved in the United States for reducing the incidence of infection in patients with nonmyeloid malignancies who are treated with chemotherapy. Studies showed that the once-per-cycle administration of pegfilgrastim compared favorably with filgrastim for the management of chemotherapy-induced neutropenia.[58]

Plerixafor has recently received FDA approval for patients who poorly mobilize autologous stem cells using traditional approaches (G-CSF and/or chemotherapy). Plerixafor is a small bicyclam molecule that reversibly and selectively antagonizes the CXCR4 chemokine receptor. Subsequently, the cognate ligand, stromal cell-derived factor-1- (CXCL12) is blocked from its target, resulting in mobilization of CD34+ cells to the peripheral blood. Plerixafor as a single agent has also been shown to mobilize stem cells comparably to traditional G-CSF for both patients and healthy donors. However, due to expense and similar mobilization of peripheral blood stem cell compared to G-CSF, the role of plerixafor as a single agent is still being established.[59]

Other Growth Factors

Additional growth factors have yet to find a consistent place in HSC transplantation. Oprelvekin (recombinant human Interleukin-11; Neumega, Genetics Institute, Cambridge, MA), currently licensed by the FDA, promotes megakaryocytopoiesis; however, it remains costly and has not been integrated into routine use for

HSC transplantation.[60] A truncated polyethylene glycol derivative preparation of thrombopoietin, megakaryocyte growth and development factor has been studied for its ability to increase circulating platelet counts in thrombocytopenic patients and plateletpheresis donors.[61] However, the development of neutralizing antibodies and iatrogenic thrombocytopenia has resulted in the closure of clinical trials.[62] Other preparations of this growth factor with thrombopoietic activity have shown efficacy in the treatment of immune thrombocytopenia and are under investigation in other settings.[61]

Nonmyeloablative HPC Transplantation

Traditionally, standard marrow transplant protocols depended on high-dose chemotherapy to eliminate the patient's cancer cells and to prepare the marrow for donor cell engraftment. However, newer protocols involve transplants with lower doses of irradiation and lower doses of chemotherapy without total marrow ablation.[63] Nonmyeloablative HPC transplantations are performed to enhance the graft-vs-leukemia effect while minimizing transplant-related morbidity and mortality. They also permit transplantation of older patients. DLIs may also be used after a nonmyeloablative HPC transplantation to boost the recipient's immune system and enhance the antitumor effect.[64]

Patients do not experience the same peritransplant toxicity, pancytopenia, and infection risks with nonmyeloablative HPC transplants as they do with conventional myeloablative transplants. However, nonmyeloablative HPC transplantation is associated with a greater risk of low-grade GVHD; this risk does not include severe acute or chronic GVHD complications.[65] After nonmyeloablative transplantation, some patients may remain in a mixed patient-donor chimeric state. The long-term effects on recipients of a mixed chimeric marrow are unknown.

Dendritic Cells in HPC Transplantation

Dendritic cells (DCs) are antigen-presenting cells that originate from marrow and have a central role in initiating and modulating the immune response. Two types of DCs have been described; myeloid DCs and lymphoid or plasmacytoid DCs. After HPC transplantation, persistent immune suppression with infectious complication risks may involve DCs. In addition, studies showed that the occurrence of GVHD and relapse may involve the DC system.[66] Further studies in this area will better define the role of DCs after HPC transplantation.[67] Recently, autologous DCs activated by recombinant prostatic acid phosphatase have been approved by the FDA for the treatment of hormone refractory metastatic prostate cancer (Sipuleucel-T, Provenge, Dendreon, Seattle, WA).

Transfusion Therapy in HPC Transplantation

Before transplantation, all cellular blood components should be leukocyte reduced to decrease HLA alloimmunization, CMV transmission, and febrile reactions.[68] The development of alloimmunization to histocompatibility antigens poses an increased risk for subsequent platelet transfusion refractoriness.[69] Therefore, blood component exposure should be minimized, and transfusions from potential progenitor cell donors should be particularly avoided. After transplantation, patients typically experience 2 or more weeks of marrow aplasia, during which extensive red cell and platelet support is required. The use of HPC, Apheresis and hematopoietic growth factors have shortened this interval and reduced the requirement for transfusion support. In contrast, cord blood transplants are frequently associated with a prolonged need for platelet support.[38] If ABO differences between donor and recipient exist, the patient's blood group will change, and careful planning is required. Such ABO mismatches can be major (eg, transplant from a group A donor to a group O patient) or minor (eg, transplant from a group O donor to a group A patient). In major mismatches, the recipient is at risk for severe intravascular hemolysis of red cells in the marrow graft; this can be prevented by erythrocyte depletion of the graft before transplant (see Table 9 for transfusion support).[70] In HPC, Apheresis transplants, the red cell content is sufficiently low (<50 mL) that red cell depletion is not usually required. Additional complications include delayed red cell engraftment and late hemolysis of engrafted donor red cells at 40 to 60 days after transplantation, as a result of residual host anti-A or -B.[71] Similar problems may be encountered if the recipient has a clinically relevant alloantibody to an antigen expressed on the donor's red cells. At the time of infusion, the immediate hazards of minor mismatches can be avoided by depleting the graft of incompatible plasma. However, engrafted donor lymphocytes may produce antibodies against recipient red cell antigens, which can result in massive fatal hemolysis of residual recipient red cells 1 to 3 weeks after transplantation.[72-74] Massive hemolysis after minor ABO-mismatched HPC transplants is associated with single-agent cyclosporine GVHD prophylaxis in patients not receiving posttransplant methotrexate.[75] For these reasons, a blood bank consultation should be obtained to assess the clinical implications of any patient receiving a red cell mismatched transplant. Both pre- and posttransplant transfusion therapy should be planned in close cooperation with the blood bank. A practical transfusion guideline for ABO-mismatched allogeneic transplantation is provided in Table 9.

In summary, for ABO-mismatched grafts, the transfusion service supplies RBCs and plasma that are compatible with both the donor's and the recipient's blood types. All transplant recipients are profoundly immunosuppressed and thus at risk for fatal TA-GVHD after transfusions of cellular blood components. Consequently, all such transfusion units must be irradiated (25 Gy or 2500 cGy) before use. Transplant recipients are also at risk for hematopoietic transplant-associated GVHD, which is caused by the engraftment of lymphocytes contained in the progenitor cell

Table 9. Transfusion Support for Patients Undergoing ABO-Mismatched Allogeneic HPC Transplantation

Recipient	Donor	Mismatch Type	Phase I All Components	RBCs	Phase II First Choice Platelets	Next Choice Platelets*	FFP	Phase III All Components
A	O	Minor	Recipient	O	A	AB; B; O	A, AB	Donor
B	O	Minor	Recipient	O	B	AB; A; O	B, AB	Donor
AB	O	Minor	Recipient	O	AB	A; B; O	AB	Donor
AB	A	Minor	Recipient	A	AB	A; B; O	AB	Donor
AB	B	Minor	Recipient	B	AB	B; A; O	AB	Donor
O	A	Major	Recipient	O	A	AB; B; O	A, AB	Donor
O	B	Major	Recipient	O	B	AB; A; O	B, AB	Donor
O	AB	Major	Recipient	O	AB	A; B; O	AB	Donor

198

Recipient	Donor			RBCs		FFP		
A	AB	Major	Recipient	A	AB	A; B; O	AB	Donor
B	AB	Major	Recipient	B	AB	B; A; O	AB	Donor
A	B	Minor and major	Recipient	O	AB	A; B; O	AB	Donor
B	A	Minor and major	Recipient	O	AB	B; A; O	AB	Donor

HPC = hematopoietic progenitor cell; FFP = Fresh Frozen Plasma; RBCs = Red Blood Cells. Phase I = from the time when the patient/recipient is prepared for HPC transplantation; Phase II = from the initiation of myeloablative therapy until direct antiglobulin test is negative and antidonor isohemagglutinins are no longer detectable (ie, the reverse typing is donor type) (for RBCs) or until recipient's erythrocytes are no longer detectable (ie, the forward typing is consistent with donor's ABO group) (for FFP); Phase III = after the forward and reverse type of the patient are consistent with donor's ABO group. Beginning from Phase I, all cellular components should be irradiated and leukocyte reduced.

*Platelet concentrates should be selected in the order presented.

product. GVHD occurs commonly after allogeneic transplantation and is generally treatable. The incidence of chronic, rather than acute, GVHD is greater after apheresis graft transplantation than after marrow graft transplantation, presumably because of the higher content of T cells in apheresis collections.[25] T-cell depletion, typically to $<10^5$ T cells/kg, has been used to reduce the incidence of GVHD but at the expense of increased graft failure, infection rate, and relapse. The progenitor cell product must *never* be irradiated, as this would prevent engraftment.

CMV infection may develop after HPC transplantation and is associated with high morbidity. The risk of infection is influenced most by the CMV serologic status of the recipient before transplantation.[76] Cellular blood component (or HPC) transfusions from CMV-seropositive donors to CMV-seronegative recipients may lead to seroconversion and symptomatic infection. Seropositive transplant recipients may experience reactivation of latent CMV infection, regardless of donor CMV exposure. Although newer therapeutic advances (eg, gancyclovin) may reduce the incidence and severity of CMV infection, all CMV-seronegative transplant patients should receive cellular blood components that are CMV seronegative or leukocytereduced.[77,78]

Autologous HPC transplantation is associated with fewer transfusion-related hazards. The donor and recipient are, by definition, ABO- and HLA-identical. Although the degree of posttransplant immunosuppression is reduced, all cellular blood components (except the transplant itself) must nevertheless be irradiated. CMV-seronegative patients should receive CMV-reduced-risk cellular components.

References

1. Zubair AC, Silberstein L, Ritz J. Adult hematopoietic stem cell plasticity. Transfusion 2002;42:1096-101.
2. Wiseman DH. Donor cell leukemia: A review. Biol Blood Marrow Transplant 2011;17:771-89.

3. Krause DS, Theise ND, Collector MI, et al. Multi-organ, multi-lineage engraftment by a single bone marrow-derived stem cell. Cell 2001;105:369-77.

4. Phinney DG, Prockop DJ. Concise review. Mesenchymal stem/multipotent stromal cells: The state of transdifferentiation and modes of tissue repair—current views. Stem Cells 2007;25:2896-902.

5. Treleaven JG, Mehta J. Bone marrow and peripheral blood stem cell harvesting. J Hematother 1992;1:215-23.

6. AABB, AATB, ARC, ASBMT, ASFA, FACT, ICCBA, ISCT, NMDP. Circular of information for the use of cellular therapy products. Bethesda, MD: AABB, 2005 (Available at http://www.aabb.org.)

7. Kao GS, Kim HT, Daley H, et al. Validation of short-term handling and storage conditions for marrow and peripheral blood stem cell products. Transfusion 2011;51:137-47.

8. Blume KG, Forman SJ, Appelbaum FR. Thomas' hematopoietic cell transplantation. 3rd ed. Malden, MA: Wiley-Blackwell, 2004:588-98.

9. Rowley SD. Hematopoietic stem cell transplantation between red cell incompatible donor-recipient pairs. Bone Marrow Transplant 2001;28:315-21.

10. Miller JP, Perry EH, Price TH, et al. Recovery and safety profiles of marrow and PBSC donor: Experience of the National Marow Donor Program. Biol Blood Marrow Transplant 2008;14(9 Suppl):29-36.

11. National Marrow Donor Program Standards. 20th ed. Minneapolis, MN: National Marrow Donor Program, 2009.

12. Parkkali T, Juvonen E, Volin L, et al. Collection of autologous blood for bone marrow donation: How useful is it? Bone Marrow Transplant 2005;35:1035-9.

13. Calmels B, Lemarie L, Esterni B, et al. Occurrence and severity of adverse events after autologous hematopoietic progenitor cell infusion are related to the amount of granulocytes in the apheresis product. Transfusion 2007;47:1268-75.

14. Cooling L, Gorlin JB. Transfusion reactions associated with hematopoietic progenitor cell reinfusion. In: Popovsky MA, ed. Transfusion reactions. 3rd ed. Bethesda, MD: AABB Press, 2007:301-30.

15. Davis-Sproul J, Haley NR, McMannis JD. Collecting and processing marrow products for transplantation. In: Roback JD, Combs MR, Grossman BJ, Hillyer CD, eds. Core principles in cellular therapy. Bethesda, MD: AABB, 2008:1-24.

16. Mavroudis D, Read E, Cottler-Fox M, et al. CD34+ cell dose predicts survival, posttransplant morbidity, and rate of hematologic recovery after allogeneic marrow transplants for hematologic malignancies. Blood 1996;88:3223-9.

17. Padley D, ed. Standards for cellular therapy product services. 3rd ed. Bethesda, MD: AABB, 2008.

18. Haas R, Mohle R, Fruhauf S, et al. Patient characteristics associated with successful mobilizing and autografting of peripheral blood progenitor cells in malignant lymphoma. Blood 1994;83:3787-94.

19. Meisenberg B, Brehm T, Schmeckel A, et al. A combination of low-dose cyclophosphamide and colony-stimulating factors is more cost-effective than granulocyte-colony-stimulating factors alone in mobilizing peripheral blood stem and progenitor cells. Transfusion 1998;38:209-15.

20. Morton J, Morton A, Bird R, et al. Predictors for optimal mobilization and subsequent engraftment of peripheral blood progenitor cells following intermediate dose cyclophosphamide and G-CSF. Leuk Res 1997;21:21-7.

21. Moskowitz CH, Glassman JR, Wuest D, et al. Factors affecting mobilization of peripheral blood progenitor cells in patients with lymphoma. Clin Cancer Res 1998;4:311-6.

22. Bolan CD, Carter CS, Wesley RA, et al. Prospective evaluation of cell kinetics, yields and donor experiences during a single large-volume apheresis versus two smaller volume consecutive day collections of allogeneic peripheral blood stem cells. Br J Haematol 2003;120:801-7.

23. Stroncek DF, Confer DL, Leitman SF. Peripheral blood progenitor cells for HPC transplants involving unrelated donors. Transfusion 2000;40:731-41.
24. Gertz MA. Current status of stem cell mobilization. Br J Haematol 2010;150:647-62.
25. Stem Cell Trialists' Collaborative Group. Allogeneic peripheral blood stem-cell compared with bone marrow transplantation in the management of hematologic malignancies: An individual patient data meta-analysis of nine randomized trials. J Clin Oncol 2005;23:5074-87.
26. Mohle R, Kanz L. Hematopoietic growth factors for hematopoietic stem cell mobilization and expansion. Semin Hematol 2007;44:193-202.
27. Favre G, Beksac M, Bacigalupo A, et al. Differences between graft product and donor side effects following bone marrow or stem cell donation. Bone Marrow Transplant 2003;32:873-80.
28. Anderlini P, Champlin RE. Biologic and molecular effects of granulocyte colony-stimulating factor in normal individuals: Recent findings and current challenges. Blood 2007; 111:1767-72.
29. McCullough J, Kahn J, Adamson J, et al. Hematopoietic growth factors—use in normal blood and stem cell donors: Clinical and ethical issues. Transfusion 2008;48:25-30.
30. Iannalfi A, Bambi F, Tintori V, et al. Peripheral blood progenitor uncontrolled-rate freezing: A single pediatric center experience. Transfusion 2007;47:2202-6.
31. Peters C, Cornish JM, Parikh, SH, et al. Stem cell source and outcome after hematopoietic stem cell transplantation (HSCT) in children and adolescents with acute leukemia. Pediatr Clin North Am 2010;57:27-46.
32. Gluckman E, Broxmeyer HA, Auerbach AD, et al. Hematopoietic reconstitution in a patient with Fanconi's anemia by means of umbilical-cord blood from an HLA-identical sibling. N Engl J Med 1989;321:1174-8.
33. Gluckman E, Rocha V, Boyer-Chammard A, et al. Outcome of cord-blood transplantation from related and unre-

lated donors. Eurocord Transplant Group and the European Blood and Marrow Transplantation Group. N Engl J Med 1997;337:373-81.

34. Escalon MP, Komanduri KV. Cord blood transplantation: Evolving strategies to improve engraftment and immune reconstitution. Curr Opin Oncol 2010;22:122-9.

35. Wagner JE, Broxmeyer HE, Cooper S. Umbilical cord and placental blood hematopoietic stem cells: Collection, cryopreservation, and storage. J Hematother 1992;1:167-73.

36. Kurtzberg J, Laughlin M, Graham ML, et al. Placental blood as a source of hematopoietic stem cells for transplantation into unrelated recipients. N Engl J Med 1996;335:157-66.

37. Brunstein CG, Barker JN, Weisdorf DJ, et al. Umbilical cord blood transplantation after nonmyeloablative conditioning: Impact on transplantation outcomes in 110 adults with hematologic disease. Blood 2007;110:3064-70.

38. Rubinstein P, Carrier C, Scaradavou A, et al. Outcomes among 562 recipients of placental-blood transplants from unrelated donors. N Engl J Med 1998;339:1565-77.

39. Kurtzberg J, Lyerly AD, Sugarman J. Untying the Gordian knot: Policies, practices, and ethical issues related to banking of umbilical cord blood. J Clin Invest 2005;115:2592-7.

40. Kao IT, Yao CL, Kong ZL, et al. Generation of natural killer cells from serum-free, expanded human umbilical cord blood CD34(+) cells. Stem Cells Dev 2007;16:1043-51.

41. Deol A, Lum LG. Role of donor lymphocyte infusions in relapsed hematological malignancies after stem cell transplantation revisited. Cancer Treat Rev 2010;36:528-38.

42. Alyea E, Weller E, Schlossman R, et al. T-cell-depleted allogeneic bone marrow transplantation followed by donor lymphocyte infusion in patients with multiple myeloma: Induction of graft-versus-myeloma effect. Blood 2001;98:934-9.

43. Fozza C, Szydlo RM, Abdel-Rehim MM, et al. Factors for graft-versus-host disease after donor lymphocyte infusions with an escalating dose regimen: Lack of association with cell dose. Br J Haematol 2007;136:833-6.

44. Atluri S, Neville K, Davis M, et al. Epstein-Barr-associated leiomyomatosis and T-cell chimerism after haploidentical bone marrow transplantation for severe combined immunodeficiency disease. J Pediatr Hematol Oncol 2007;29:166-72.

45. Goodnough LT, Anderson KC. Recombinant growth factors. Transfus Sci 1995;16:45-62.

46. Klingemann HG, Shepherd JD, Eaves CJ, Eaves AC. The role of erythropoietin and other growth factors in transfusion medicine. Transfus Med Rev 1991;5:33-47.

47. Fischl M, Galpin JE, Levine JD, et al. Recombinant human erythropoietin for patients with AIDS treated with zidovudine. N Engl J Med 1990;322:1488-93.

48. Demetri GD, Kris M, Wade J, et al. Quality-of-life benefit in chemotherapy patients treated with epoetin alfa is independent of disease response or tumor type: Results from a prospective community oncology study. Procrit Study Group. J Clin Oncol 1998;16:3412-25.

49. Corwin HL, Gettinger A, Fabian TC, et al. Efficacy and safety of epoetin alfa in critically ill patients. N Engl J Med 2007;357:965-76.

50. Singh AK, Szczech L, Tang KL, et al. Correction of anemia with epoetin alfa in chronic kidney disease. N Engl J Med 2006;355:2085-98.

51. Fishbane S, Nissenson AR. The new FDA label for erythropoietin treatment: How does it affect hemoglobin target? Kidney Int 2007;72:806-13.

52. Rizzo JD, Somerfield MR, Hagerty KL, et al. Use of epoetin and darbepoetin in patients with cancer: 2007. American Society of Hematology/American Society of Clinical Oncology clinical practice guideline update. Blood 2008; 111:25-41.

53. Macdougall IC, Gray SJ, Elston O, et al. Pharmacokinetics of novel erythropoiesis stimulating protein compared with epoetin alfa in dialysis patients. J Am Soc Nephrol 1999;10:2392-5.

54. Smith TJ, Khatcheressian J, Lyman GH, et al. 2006 update of recommendations for the use of white blood cell growth factors: An evidence-based clinical practice guideline. J Clin Oncol 2006;24:3187-205.

55. Ottmann OG, Bug G, Krauter J. Current status of growth factors in the treatment of acute myeloid and lymphoblastic leukemia. Semin Hematol 2007;44:183-92.

56. Strauss RG. Neutrophil (granulocyte) transfusions in the new millennium. Transfusion 1998;38:710-12.

57. Freedman MH. Safety of long-term administration of granulocyte colony-stimulating factor for severe chronic neutropenia. Curr Opin Hematol 1997;4:217-24.

58. Crawford J. Once-per-cycle pegfilgrastim (Neulasta) for the management of chemotherapy-induced neutropenia. Semin Oncol 2003;30:24-30.

59. Mohty M, Duarte RF, Croockewit S, et al. The role of plerixafor in optimizing peripheral blood stem cell mobilization for autologous stem cell transplantation. Leukemia 2011;25:1-6.

60. Bhatia M, Davenport V, Cairo MS. The role of interleukin-11 to prevent chemotherapy-induced thrombocytopenia in patients with solid tumors, lymphoma, acute myeloid leukemia and bone marrow failure syndromes. Leuk Lymphoma 2007;48:9-15.

61. Kuter DJ. New thrombopoietic growth factors. Blood 2007;109:4607-16.

62. Li J, Yang C, Xia Y, et al. Thrombocytopenia caused by the development of antibodies to thrombopoietin. Blood 2001;98:3241-8.

63. Mielcarek M, Storer BE, Sandmaier BM, et al. Comparable outcomes after nonmyeloablative hematopoietic cell transplantation with unrelated and related donors. Biol Blood Marrow Transplant 2007;13:1499-507.

64. Childs R, Chernoff A, Contentin N, et al. Regression of metastatic renal-cell carcinoma after nonmyeloablative allogeneic peripheral-blood stem-cell transplantation. N Engl J Med 2000;343:750-8.
65. Sala-Torra O, Martin PJ, Storer B, et al. Serious acute or chronic graft-versus-host disease after hematopoietic cell transplantation: A comparison of myeloablative and non-myeloablative conditioning regimens. Bone Marrow Transplant 2008;41:887-93.
66. Mohty M. Dendritic cells and acute graft-versus-host disease after allogeneic stem cell transplantation. Leuk Lymphoma 2007;48:1696-701.
67. Morelli AE, Thomson AW. Tolerogenic dendritic cells and the quest for transplant tolerance. Nat Rev Immunol 2007; 7:610-21.
68. Szczepiorkowski Z. Transfusion support for hematopoietic transplant recipients. In: Roback JD, Combs MR, Grossman BJ, Hillyer CD, eds. Core principles in cellular therapy. Bethesda, MD: AABB, 2008:73-90.
69. Slichter SJ. Platelet transfusion therapy. Hematol Oncol Clin North Am 2007;21:697-729.
70. Larghero J, Rea D, Esperou H, et al. ABO-mismatched marrow processing for transplantation: Results of 114 procedures and analysis of immediate adverse events and hematopoietic recovery. Transfusion 2006;46:398-402.
71. Griffith LM, McCoy JP Jr, Bolan CD, et al. Persistence of recipient plasma cells and anti-donor isohaemagglutinins in patients with delayed donor erythropoiesis after major ABO incompatible non-myeloablative haematopoietic cell transplantation. Br J Haematol 2005;128:668-75.
72. Bolan CD, Childs RW, Procter JL, et al. Massive immune haemolysis after allogeneic peripheral blood stem cell transplantation with minor ABO incompatibility. Br J Haematol 2001;112:787-95.
73. Laurencet FM, Samii K, Bressoud A, et al. Massive delayed hemolysis following peripheral blood stem cell

transplantation with minor ABO incompatibility. Hematol Cell Ther 1997;39:159-62.

74. Reed M, Yearsley M, Krugh D, Kennedy MS. Severe hemolysis due to passenger lymphocyte syndrome after hematopoietic stem cell transplantation from an HLA-matched related donor. Arch Pathol Lab Med 2003;127: 1366-8.

75. Gajewski JL, Petz LD, Calhoun L, et al. Hemolysis of transfused group O red blood cells in minor ABO-incompatible unrelated-donor bone marrow transplants in patients receiving cyclosporine without posttransplant methotrexate. Blood 1992;79:3076-85.

76. Ganepola S, Gentilini C, Hilbers U, et al. Patients at high risk for CMV infection and disease show delayed CD8+ T-cell immune recovery after allogeneic stem cell transplantation. Bone Marrow Transplant 2007;39:293-9.

77. Bowden RA, Slichter SJ, Sayers M, et al. A comparison of filtered leukocyte-reduced and cytomegalovirus (CMV) seronegative blood products for the prevention of transfusion-associated CMV infection after marrow transplant. Blood 1995;86:3598-603.

78. Nichols WG, Price TH, Gooley T, et al. Transfusion-transmitted cytomegalovirus infection after receipt of leukoreduced blood products. Blood 2003;101:4195-200.

THERAPEUTIC APHERESIS

Description

Therapeutic apheresis involves the separation of a patient's whole blood to remove and in many cases, to replace a whole blood component that contains an abnormal constituent, in order to achieve a clinical benefit.[1] Specific procedures are defined by the blood component removed: cytapheresis (any cellular element) including leukapheresis, lymphocytapheresis, erythrocytapheresis and plateletpheresis, or therapeutic plasma exchange (TPE).[2] Although several of these procedures can be performed manually, the use of automated cell separators permits the processing of larger quantities of blood safely. It also allows more efficient component removal and the simultaneous reinfusion of remaining blood constituents with replacement of the removed component.

The American Society for Apheresis (ASFA) and AABB have categorized the evidence for the efficacy of therapeutic apheresis with respect to various diseases. The Apheresis Applications Committee of ASFA published the most recent iteration of their indications for therapeutic apheresis using an evidence-based approach.[3] Adopting the University HealthSystem Consortium evidence quality criteria, ASFA developed a fact sheet format for each disease treated by apheresis indicating the strength of evidence and its treatment category. The ASFA Journal of Clinical Apheresis Special Issue (fifth edition) has further improved the process of using evidence-based medicine in the recommendations by refining the category definitions and by adding a grade of recommendation based on the widely accepted GRADE system (Grading of Recommendations Assessment, Development and Evaluation). Table 10 contains abbreviated principles of grading recommendations derived from Guyatt et al.[4]

ASFA Category I defines diseases for which therapeutic apheresis is first-line therapy, either as a primary stand-alone treatment or in conjunction with other modes of treatment. Category II defines diseases for which therapeutic apheresis is generally accepted as second-line therapy, either as a stand-alone treatment or in conjunction with other modes of treatment. Category III includes diseases where the optimal role of apheresis therapy is not established and decision making should be individualized. Category IV includes diseases for which published evidence demonstrates or suggests apheresis to be ineffective or harmful. Institutional Review Board approval is desirable if apheresis treatment is undertaken in these circumstances. Table 11 categorizes the most common diseases treated by therapeutic apheresis.

Indications

Cytapheresis

Therapeutic cytapheresis can be used to reduce either excessive or abnormal cellular elements in the blood. This technique is typically employed in emergency situations when conventional therapies are ineffective or slow to take effect. The resulting post-procedure improvement is temporary and may, or may not, affect long-term clinical outcome.

Erythrocytapheresis or red cell exchange by apheresis has been used to manage acute severe sickle cell disease crises such as stroke and acute chest syndrome, by reducing the level of hemoglobin S to less than 30%. For long-term stroke prophylaxis, reducing the level of hemoglobin S to less than 30% to

Table 10. Grading Recommendations*

Recommendation	Description	Methodological Quality of Supporting Evidence	Implications
Grade 1A	strong recommendation, high-quality evidence	RCTs without important limitations or overwhelming evidence from observational studies	Strong recommendation, can apply to most patients in most circumstances without reservation
Grade 1B	strong recommendation, moderate quality evidence	RCTs with important limitations (inconsistent results, methodological flaws, indirect, or imprecise) or exceptionally strong evidence from observational studies	Strong recommendation, can apply to most patients in most circumstances without reservation
Grade 1C	strong recommendation, low-quality or very low-quality evidence	Observational studies or case series	Strong recommendation but may change when higher quality evidence becomes available

(Continued)

Table 10. Grading Recommendations* (Continued)

Recommendation	Description	Methodological Quality of Supporting Evidence	Implications
Grade 2A	weak recommendation, high quality evidence	RCTs without important limitations or overwhelming evidence from observational studies	Weak recommendation, best action may differ depending on circumstances or patients' or societal values
Grade 2B	weak recommendation, moderate-quality evidence	RCTs with important limitations (inconsistent results, methodological flaws, indirect, or imprecise) or exceptionally strong evidence from observational studies	Weak recommendation, best action may differ depending on circumstances or patients' or societal values
Grade 2C	weak recommendation, low-quality or very low-quality evidence	Observational studies or case series	Very weak recommendations; other alternatives may be equally reasonable

*Adapted from Guyatt G, Gutterman D, Baumann MH, Addrizzo-Harris D, Hylek EM, Phillips B, Raskob G, Lewis SZ, Schunemann H. Grading strength of recommendations and quality of evidence in clinical guidelines: report from an American College of Chest physicians task force. Chest 2006;129:174-81.

Table 11. ASFA 2010 Indication Categories for Therapeutic Apheresis*

Disease Name	Special Condition	TA Modality	Category	Recommendation Grade
ABO-incompatible hematopoietic stem cell transplantation	HPC, Marrow	TPE	II	1B
	HPC, Apheresis	TPE	II	2B
ABO-incompatible solid organ transplantation	Kidney	TPE	II	1B
	Heart (<40 months of age)	TPE	II	1C
	Liver perioperative	TPE	III	2C
Acute disseminated encephalomyelitis		TPE	II	2C
Acute inflammatory demyelinating polyneuropathy (Guillain-Barré syndrome)		TPE	I	1A
Acute liver failure		TPE	III	2B
Age-related macular degeneration (AMD)	Dry AMD	Rheopheresis	III	2B

(Continued)

213

Table 11. ASFA 2010 Indication Categories for Therapeutic Apheresis* (Continued)

Disease Name	Special Condition	TA Modality	Category	Recommendation Grade
Amyloidosis, systemic		TPE	IV	2C
Amyotrophic lateral sclerosis		TPE	IV	1B
ANCA-associated rapidly progressive glomerulonephritis (Wegener granulomatosis)	Dialysis dependence	TPE	I	1A
	Diffuse alveolar hemorrhage (DAH)	TPE	I	1C
	Dialysis independence	TPE	III	2C
Antiglomerular basement membrane disease (Goodpasture syndrome)	Dialysis independence	TPE	I	1A
	Diffuse alveolar hemorrhage	TPE	I	1B
	Dialysis-dependent and no DAH	TPE	IV	1A
Aplastic anemia; pure red cell aplasia	Aplastic anemia	TPE	III	2C
	Pure red cell aplasia	TPE	II	2C

Autoimmunic hemolytic anemia: warm autoimmune hemolytic anemia; cold agglutinin disease	Warm autoimmune hemolytic anemia	TPE	III	2C
	Cold agglutinin disease (life-threatening)	TPE	II	2C
Babesiosis	Severe	RBC exchange	I	1B
	High-risk population	RBC exchange	II	2C
Burn shock resuscitation		TPE	IV	2B
Cardiac allograft rejection	Prophylaxis	ECP	I	1A
	Treatment of rejection	ECP	II	1B
	Treatment of antibody-mediated rejection	TPE	III	2C
Catastrophic antiphospholipid syndrome		TPE	II	2C
Chronic focal encephalitis (Rasmussen's encephalitis)		TPE	II	2C
		IA	II	2C

(Continued)

Table 11. ASFA 2010 Indication Categories for Therapeutic Apheresis* (Continued)

Disease Name	Special Condition	TA Modality	Category	Recommen-dation Grade
Chronic inflammatory demyeli-nating polyradiculoneuro-pathy		TPE	I	1B
Coagulation factor inhibitors		IA	III	2B
		TPE	IV	2C
Cryoglobulinemia	Severe/symptomatic	TPE	I	1B
	Secondary to hepatitis C virus	IA	II	2B
Cutaneous T-cell lymphoma; mycosis fungoides; Sézary syndrome	Erythrodermic	ECP	I	1B
	Non-erythrodermic	ECP	III	2C
Dermatomyositis or polymyo-sitis		TPE	IV	1B
		Leukocytapheresis	IV	1B
Dilated cardiomyopathy	NYHA II-IV	IA	III	2B
	NYHA II-IV	TPE	III	2C

Familial hypercholesterolemia	Homozygotes	Selective removal	I	1A
	Heterozygotes	Selective removal	II	1A
	Homozygotes with small blood volume	TPE	II	1C
Focal segmental glomerulosclerosis recurrent		TPE	I	1C
Graft-vs-host disease	Skin (chronic)	ECP	II	1B
	Skin (acute)	ECP	II	2C
	Non-skin (acute/chronic)	ECP	III	2C
Hereditary hemochromatosis		Erythrocytapheresis	III	2B
Hemolytic uremic syndrome (HUS)	Atypical HUS due to complement factor gene mutations	TPE	II	2C
	Atypical HUS due to autoantibody to factor H	TPE	I	2C
	Diarrhea-associated HUS or typical HUS	TPE	IV	1C

(Continued)

Table 11. ASFA 2010 Indication Categories for Therapeutic Apheresis* (Continued)

Disease Name	Special Condition	TA Modality	Category	Recommendation Grade
Hyperleukocytosis	Leukostasis	Leukocytapheresis	I	1B
	Prophylaxis	Leukocytapheresis	III	2C
Hypertriglyceridemic pancreatitis		TPE	III	2C
Hyperviscosity in monoclonal gammopathies	Treatment of symptoms	TPE	I	1B
	Prophylaxis for rituximab	TPE	I	1C
Immune thrombocytopenia		TPE	IV	1C
Immune complex rapidly progressive glomerulonephritis		TPE	III	2B
Inclusion body myositis		TPE	IV	2B
		Leukocytapheresis	IV	2C
Inflammatory bowel disease		Adsorptive cytapheresis	II	2B

Lambert-Eaton myasthenic syndrome		TPE	II	2C
Lung allograft rejection		ECP	II	1C
Malaria	Severe	RBC exchange	II	2B
Multiple sclerosis	Acute CNS inflammatory demyelinating disease unresponsive to steroids	TPE	II	1B
	Chronic progressive	TPE	III	2B
Myasthenia gravis	Moderate-severe	TPE	I	1A
	Pre-thymectomy	TPE	I	1C
Myeloma cast nephropathy	Cast nephropathy	TPE	II	2B
Nephrogenic systemic fibrosis		ECP	III	2C
		TPE	III	2C
Neuromyelitis optica (Devic syndrome)		TPE	II	1C

(Continued)

Table 11. ASFA 2010 Indication Categories for Therapeutic Apheresis* (Continued)

Disease Name	Special Condition	TA Modality	Category	Recommen-dation Grade
Overdose, venoms, and poisoning	Mushroom poisoning	TPE	II	2C
	Invenomation	TPE	III	2C
	Monoclonal antibody with PML	TPE	III	2C
	Other compounds	TPE	III	2C
Paraneoplastic neurologic syndromes		TPE	III	2C
		IA	III	2C
Paraproteinemic polyneuro-pathies	IgG/IgA	TPE	I	1B
	IgM	TPE	I	1C
	Multiple myeloma	TPE	III	2C
	IgG/IgA or IgM	IA	III	2C

Pediatric autoimmune neuropsychiatric disorders associated with streptococcal infections (PANDAS) and Sydenham chorea	PANDAS (exacerbation)	TPE	I	1B
	Sydenham chorea	TPE	I	1B
Pemphigus vulgaris		TPE	IV	2B
		ECP	III	2C
Phytanic acid storage disease (Refsum disease)		TPE	II	2C
Polycythemia vera and erythrocytosis	Polycythemia vera	Erythrocytapheresis	III	2C
	Secondary erythrocytosis	Erythrocytapheresis	III	2B
POEMS (polyneuropathy, organomegaly, endocrinopathy, M protein, and skin changes)		TPE	IV	2B
Posttransfusion purpura		TPE	III	2C
Psoriasis		TPE	IV	1B

(Continued)

Table 11. ASFA 2010 Indication Categories for Therapeutic Apheresis* (Continued)

Disease Name	Special Condition	TA Modality	Category	Recommen-dation Grade
Red cell alloimmunization in pregnancy	Prior to intrauterine transfusion availability	TPE	II	2C
Renal transplantation	Antibody-mediated rejection	TPE	I	1B
	Desensitization, living donor, positive crossmatch due to donor specific HLA antibody	TPE	II	1B
	High PRA; cadaveric donor	TPE	III	2C
Rheumatoid arthritis, refractory		IA	II	2A
		TPE	IV	1B
Schizophrenia		TPE	IV	1A
Scleroderma (Progressive systemic sclerosis)		TPE	III	2C
		ECP	IV	1A
Sepsis with multi-organ failure		TPE	III	2B
Sickle cell disease	Acute stroke	RBC exchange	I	1C

	Acute chest syndrome	RBC exchange	II	1C
	Prophylaxis for primary or secondary stroke; prevention of transfusional iron overload	RBC exchange	II	1C
	Multi-organ failure	RBC exchange	III	2C
Stiff-person syndrome		TPE	IV	2C
Systemic lupus erythematosus	Severe (eg, cerebritis, diffuse alveolar hemorrhage)	TPE	II	2C
	Nephritis	TPE	IV	1B
Thrombocytosis	Symptomatic	Thrombocytapheresis	II	2C
	Prophylactic or secondary	Thrombocytapheresis	III	2C
Thrombotic microangiopathy: drug-associated	Ticlopidine/Clopidogrel	TPE	I	2B
	Cyclosporine/Tacrolimus	TPE	III	2C
	Gemcitabine	TPE	IV	2C
	Quinine	TPE	IV	2B

(Continued)

Table 11. ASFA 2010 Indication Categories for Therapeutic Apheresis* (Continued)

Disease Name	Special Condition	TA Modality	Category	Recommendation Grade
Thrombotic microangiopathy: hematopoietic stem cell transplant-associated		TPE	III	1B
Thrombotic thrombocytopenic purpura		TPE	I	1A
Thyroid storm		TPE	III	2C
Wilson disease, fulminant	Fulminant hepatic failure with hemolysis	TPE	I	1C

*Modified from Szczepiorkowski SM et al.[3]

ASFA = American Society for Apheresis; I = standard therapy; II = secondary therapy; III = no optimal use established; IV = ineffective in controlled trials; TPE = therapeutic plasma exchange; ECP = extracorporeal photopheresis; RBC = Red Blood Cell; IA = immunoadsorption; TA = therapeutic apheresis; HPC = hematopoietic progenitor cell; NYHA = New York Heart Association; PRA = panel-reactive antibody; PML = progressive multifocal leukoencephalopathy.

50% with a chronic schedule of apheresis has been successful.[5,6] Erythrocytapheresis is effective in managing and preventing iron overload associated with chronic transfusion in patients with sickle cell disease.[7] Other indications for erythrocytapheresis are rare. It has been used to treat overwhelming parasitic infections with malaria and babesia[5] and for immune-mediated hemolysis in the transplant setting.

Cytapheresis is also useful in the management of hyperleukocytosis with leukostasis and, less frequently, thrombocytosis in patients with acute leukemia or myeloproliferative disorders. Leukostasis is characterized by central nervous system and/or pulmonary symptoms caused by excessive leukoblasts in the microcirculation. By achieving immediate, although temporary, reductions in circulating white cells, leukapheresis is typically initiated to correct life-threatening leukostasis in patients with myeloblast counts >70,000 to 100,000/μL. Cell subtype appears to be important, and symptoms appear more frequently in patients with acute myelogenous leukemia (particularly monocytic and myelomonocytic morphology) than in patients with lymphocytic leukemias or chronic myelogenous leukemia. Multiple procedures may be required in combination with cytotoxic therapy to maintain lower counts because of intravascular migration of tumor cells. The efficacy of leukocytapheresis for prevention of the tumor lysis syndrome (which may occur with aggressive chemotherapeutic regimens) is controversial, possibly because of the significant leukemia burden outside the circulation that is not accessible to removal during a cytapheresis procedure.[8]

In patients with myeloproliferative disorders and severe symptomatic thrombocytosis, plateletpheresis can be useful in the prevention of thrombotic and hemorrhagic complications by acutely lowering the platelet count. Generally, plateletpheresis is initiated when the platelet count exceeds 1,000,000/μL. The platelet count is typically transiently lowered by 30% to 50% after a single procedure.[8,9] Plateletpheresis is uncommonly required because of the effectiveness of therapeutic agents such as anagrelide, hydroxyurea, and interferon alpha, and should be reserved for patients with severe symptomatic thrombocytosis.[8]

Another form of cytapheresis known as selective leukocyte apheresis has emerged to target removal of specific subsets of leukocytes that may participate in the pathogenesis of a disease. Two selective leukocyte apheresis devices are currently in use in Europe and Asia, specifically the leukocyte adsorptive apheresis system (LCAP) and the granulocyte monocyte adsorptive apheresis system (GMA). These have been most extensively studied in the management of inflammatory bowel disease with varying results in clinical trials.[8]

Therapeutic Plasma Exchange

Plasmapheresis refers to the separation of plasma by apheresis, such as for plasma donation. However, when significant amounts of plasma are removed and replaced, the procedure is called therapeutic plasma exchange. TPE has found widespread clinical application in the management of autoimmune, hematologic, renal, metabolic, and neurologic disorders. Most plasma exchange regimens include the processing of 1.0 to 1.5 plasma volumes for each of five to six procedures performed over a 10- to 14-day period. The volume exchanged, the number, and the frequency of procedures are dependent on the disease indication.[3] The removal of large amounts of plasma necessitates concurrent replacement with colloid, crystalloid, or a combination of solutions. Albumin (5%) is the most commonly used replacement solution. However, plasma may also be used. In patients experiencing active hemorrhage or with a high risk of bleeding, such as an invasive procedure, plasma may be used as a replacement solution to avoid the dilutional coagulopathy resulting from the use of albumin or colloid replacement alone. Patients with thrombotic thrombocytopenic purpura (TTP) are treated with daily TPE using plasma as replacement until there is normalization of the platelet count and lactate dehydrogenase.[10]

Selective Removal of Plasma Components

The removal of the specific pathologic substance rather than all of the patient plasma would avoid many of the risks of frequent plasma exchanges, including dilutional coagulopathy and the depletion of beneficial immunoglobulins. Selective adsorption columns combined with apheresis technology have been used to remove only the targeted substances.

Selective Lipid Removal (Lipid Apheresis)

Lipid apheresis [low-density lipoprotein (LDL) apheresis] can be used to reduce apolipoprotein-B-containing lipoproteins including LDL and lipoprotein(a) with conservation of high-density lipoprotein.[11] Currently, the Food and Drug Administration (FDA) has approved the use of lipid apheresis for the following categories: 1) patients who are homozygotes for hypercholesterolemia and have LDL cholesterol greater than or equal to 500 mg/dL; 2) patients who are heterozygotes for hypercholesterolemia and have LDL cholesterol greater than or equal to 300 mg/dL; and 3) patients who are heterozygotes for hypercholesterolemia and have LDL cholesterol greater than or equal to 200 mg/dL and documented coronary heart disease. The latter group typically includes patients who cannot be adequately treated with lipid-reducing medications or are intolerant of their side effects. Lipid apheresis consists of plasma separation followed by adsorption of LDL onto negatively charged dextran sulfate or LDL antibody-coated sepharose beads, precipitation of LDL by negatively charged heparin, or removal of LDL by filtration. Procedures are usually performed every 2 weeks, and a single procedure can transiently lower the LDL cholesterol by 70% to 80%.[12]

Hypotension is the most common side effect in patients undergoing lipid apheresis. Patients should discontinue taking antihypertensive medication, especially angiotensin-converting enzyme (ACE) inhibitors, at least 24 hours before treatment.

Staphylococcal Protein A Immunoadsorption

Protein A derived from *Staphylococcus aureus* has been complexed to a carrier such as silica or agarose and used for the therapeutic removal of monomeric IgG (subclasses 1, 2, and 4; use for subclass 3 is less effective) and IgG-containing immune complexes after plasma separation by apheresis.[11] The staphylococcal protein A-silica (PAS) column had received approval by the FDA for the treatment of rheumatoid arthritis in patients who are refractory or intolerant to medical therapy and in patients with immune thrombocytopenia (ITP). Unfortunately, this column is no longer being manufactured.

Photopheresis

Photopheresis has been found to be efficacious in selected malignant and autoimmune disorders. The technique involves the exposure of peripheral blood leukocytes to the drug 8-methoxypsoralen. Psoralen binds to DNA in all nucleated cells and, upon stimulation with ultraviolet light, prevents DNA replication and RNA transcription, which leads to the inhibition of lymphocyte proliferation and the induction of apoptosis of treated cells. When patients undergo a photopheresis procedure, the peripheral blood leukocytes are first harvested by a leukapheresis procedure. These isolated leukocytes are exposed to psoralen followed by ultraviolet A irradiation and then reinfused to the patient. Photopheresis has become standard therapy for advanced erythrodermic forms of cutaneous T-cell lymphoma and Sezary syndrome and has shown promise in the management of some autoimmune diseases, solid organ transplant rejection, and the prevention and management of graft-vs-host disease after allogeneic hematopoietic progenitor cell transplantation.[13]

Procedural Considerations

Vascular access is an important clinical issue in apheresis patients. Whenever possible, peripheral venous access should be used because of its lower risk. Antecubital veins are preferred. Peripheral venous access must be able to accommodate the flow rate (≥1 mL/kg/minute) required during the apheresis procedure. In addition, the patient's arms must be relatively immobilized for several hours to ensure continuation of apheresis and to lower the risk of venous penetration and nerve injury. Young age, altered mental status, inability to cooperate, frequent urination, decreased muscle tone, and hyperviscosity may preclude the use of peripheral venous access. If a central line is required, internal jugular and subclavian veins are common choices of central access. Fistulas, grafts, or shunts are also ready sites of vascular access. A femoral central venous catheter lacks the risk of pneumothorax and, should bleeding occur, pressure on the entry point can be used, unlike neck and subclavian lines. Femoral lines for emergency apheresis are a reasonable option for patients with low platelet counts. Because of their anatomic location, they have a higher risk of infection and thrombosis. If central venous catheters are used for apheresis, specialized noncollapsible types (eg, dialysis catheters) must be used. Saline or heparin must be used to maintain catheter patency. Four percent citrate, such as acid-citrate-dextrose (ACD) anticoagulant solutions, may be substituted for patients with heparin allergy.

Because of the large volume removed during plasma exchange, replacement of the volume deficit is accomplished by using 5% albumin, either alone or in combination with 0.9% normal saline. During shortages of albumin, pentastarch and hetastarch have been used as replacement.[14,15] Plasma is rarely used as primary replacement during TPE because of the risk of transfusion reactions and transfusion-transmitted disease compared to albumin. However, plasma is the required replacement solution in patients with TTP, and it may be indicated for replenishing coagulation factors in other conditions to prevent dilutional coagulopathy in patients at high risk for bleeding.

Priming of the apheresis circuit with red cells may be necessary for patients weighing less than 25 kg or patients with severe anemia, because of the extracorporeal shift of red cells in the apheresis circuit, which effectively decreases the patient's intra-procedure hematocrit.

Complications of Therapeutic Apheresis

Complications of apheresis can be procedure-related, replacement component-related, or access-related. Complications related to an apheresis procedure can occur during and after apheresis.

Citrate, found in the ACD used as anticoagulant in the apheresis circuit, chelates ionized calcium temporarily to prevent coagulation factor activation in the apheresis device. One of the more common complications during apheresis is citrate-related hypocalcemia, which manifests frequently as perioral tingling, numbness, paresthesias, or muscle cramping. Rarely, severe hypocalcemia may be associated with dysrhythmias. Manifestations of hypocalcemia are more likely in large-volume procedures or procedures in which plasma is used as the replacement solution. Symptoms can be treated with oral calcium supplements or intravenous calcium replacement (calcium gluconate or calcium chloride). Citrate-related toxicity is often transient, because the liver and kidneys can metabolize citrate quickly, and it usually resolves within minutes to hours of the cessation of apheresis. Persons with liver failure may be especially susceptible to citrate toxicity as are patients who are unable to report early symptoms. Monitoring of ionized calcium may be medically prudent in these cases. Flushing and hypotension have been reported in patients taking ACE inhibitors who receive albumin replacement during standard apheresis.[16] ACE inhibitors block the degradation of bradykinins that are present in albumin solutions. It is recommended that patients discontinue taking ACE inhibitors at least 24 hours before an apheresis procedure. Rare reactions include seizures, anaphylaxis (with plasma infusions), and cardiorespiratory arrest.

Fluid shifts occurring during apheresis can lead to hypotension, volume depletion, volume overload, or vasovagal reactions. Depletion of coagulation factors may increase the risk for bleeding and, rarely, thrombosis. Dilutional coagulopathy can be mitigated by partial plasma replacement at the end of the procedure. Because of the higher risk of infection with progressive depletion of immunoglobulins with serial plasma exchange, some patients may benefit from intravenous immune globulin infusion when IgG levels are reduced below 200 mg/dL.

Concentrations of some drugs, particularly those that are protein bound (eg, antibiotics, anticoagulants, and sedatives) and immune globulin preparations may be lowered by TPE. Whenever possible, daily medications should be administered *after* TPE. To avoid erroneous laboratory results caused by hemodilution or passively acquired antibodies from donor plasma, diagnostic and/or serologic tests must be performed on pre-apheresis blood samples. Complications related to apheresis replacement components include allergic reactions, transfusion reactions, and transfusion-transmitted diseases if patients receive blood components.

Access-related complications can be seen in both peripheral and central access. Hematoma and nerve injury can occur after venipuncture. Risks associated with central catheters include infection, catheter thrombosis, air embolism, pulmonary embolism, cardiac arrhythmias, and cardiorespiratory arrest. In patients receiving apheresis in outpatient clinics, catheter care can be particularly challenging. Catheter care including dressing changes and line flushing should be arranged to reduce risks of complication and to maintain catheter patency.[17]

References

1. Weinstein R. Basic principles of therapeutic blood exchange. In: McLeod BC, Szczepiorkowski ZM, Wein-

stein R, Winters JL, eds. Apheresis: Principles and practice. 3rd ed. Bethesda, MD: AABB Press, 2010:269-94.

2. Winters JL, Gottschall J, eds. Therapeutic apheresis: A physician's handbook. 3rd ed. Bethesda, MD: AABB/ASFA, 2011.

3. Szczepiorkowski ZM,Winters JL, Bandarenko N, et al. Guidelines on the use of therapeutic apheresis in clinical practice—evidence-based approach from the apheresis applications committee of the American Society for Apheresis. 5th ed. J Clin Apher 2010;25:83-177.

4. Guyatt G, Gutterman D, Baumann MH, et al. Grading strength of recommendations and quality of evidence in clinical guidelines: Report from an American College of Chest Physicians task force. Chest 2006;129:174-81.

5. Shaz BH. Red cell exchange and other therapeutic alterations of red cell mass. In: McLeod BC, Szczepiorkowski ZM, Weinstein R, Winters JL, eds. Apheresis: Principles and practice. 3rd ed. Bethesda, MD: AABB Press, 2010: 391-410.

6. Adams RJ, McKie VC, Hsu L, et al. Prevention of a first stroke by transfusions in children with sickle cell anemia and abnormal results on transcranial Doppler ultrasonography. N Engl J Med 1998;339:5-11.

7. Kim HC, Dugan NP, Silber JH, et al. Erythrocytapheresis therapy to reduce iron overload in chronically transfused patients with sickle cell disease. Blood 1994;83:1136-42.

8. Bandarenko N, Lockhart EL. Therapeutic leukocyte and platelet depletion. In: McLeod BC, Szczepiorkowski ZM, Weinstein R, Winters JL eds. Apheresis: Principles and practice. 3rd ed. Bethesda, MD: AABB Press, 2010:251-68.

9. Klein HG. Principles of apheresis: In: Anderson KC, Ness PM, eds. Scientific basis of transfusion medicine. Philadelphia: WB Saunders, 2000:553-68.

10. Kiss JE. Therapeutic plasma exchange in hematologic diseases and dysproteinemias. In: McLeod BC, Szczepiorkowski ZM, Weinstein R, Winters JL, eds. Apheresis:

Principles and practice. 3rd ed. Bethesda, MD: AABB Press, 2010:319-47.

11. Winters JL, Pineda AA, McLeod BC, et al. Therapeutic apheresis in renal and metabolic diseases. J Clin Apher 2000;15:53-73.

12. Winters JL. Selective extraction of plasma constituents. In: McLeod BC, Szczepiorkowski ZM, Weinstein R, Winters JL, eds. Apheresis: Principles and practice. 3rd ed. Bethesda, MD: AABB Press, 2010:411-44.

13. Choi J, Foss FM. Photopheresis. In: McLeod BC, Szczepiorkowski ZM, Weinstein R, Winters JL, eds. Apheresis: Principles and practice. 3rd ed. Bethesda, MD: AABB Press, 2010:615-34.

14. Brecher ME, Owen HG, Bandarenko N. Alternatives to albumin: Starch replacement for plasma exchange. J Clin Apher 1997;12:146-53.

15. Rock G, Sutton DM, Freedman J, Nair RC. Pentastarch instead of albumin as replacement fluid for therapeutic plasma exchange. The Canadian Apheresis Group. J Clin Apher 1997;12:165-9.

16. Owen HG, Brecher ME. Atypical reactions associated with use of angiotensin-converting enzyme inhibitors and apheresis. Transfusion 1994;34:891-4.

17. Jones HG, Bandarenko N. Management of the therapeutic apheresis patient. In: McLeod BC, Price TH, Weinstein R, eds. Apheresis: Principles and practice. 2nd ed. Bethesda, MD: AABB Press, 2003:253-82.

INDEX

for exchange transfusions, 84-85

for intrauterine transfusions, 84

for urgent transfusions, 77

Blood vessels, in hemostasis, 101-102

Blood warming, 93-94, 155, 162-163

Bovine thrombin, 52

Bradykinin, 160

C

Chagas' disease, 170

Children. *See* Neonates; Pediatric transfusions

Chills, 155

Cholesterol, 227

Chronic fatigue syndrome, 170

Circulatory overload, *152,* 157-158

Citrate toxicity, 163, 230

Clopidogrel, 104, 128

Closure time, 103

Coagulation factors. *See also* specific coagulation factors
deficiencies of, 31, 109-120
inhibitors to, 115, 116-117
replacement with Cryoprecipitated AHF, 33
replacement with Plasma, 30, 31, 32
role in hemostasis, 104-106
screening tests for, 105-106
in vitro properties of, 9, *10-11*

Coagulopathy. *See* Hemostatic disorders

Colloid solutions, 55-56

Colony-stimulating factors, 186-187, 188, 193-194

Compatibility testing. *See* Pretransfusion testing

Components, blood. *See* Blood components

Conjugated estrogens, 131

Contamination, bacterial, 21-22, *149, 153,* 160-162

Cord blood, HPCs from, 189-191

Corrected count increment, 22-23, 90

Creutzfeldt-Jakob disease, 170-171

Crossmatching
platelet, 23, 24, 91, 108
in pretransfusion testing, 69, *70,* 71

Crossmatch/transfusion ratios, 68

Cryoprecipitated Antihemophilic Factor
composition and volume of, *4*
contraindications and precautions for, 34
description of, 32-33
dose and administration of, 34
indications for, *4,* 33
DIC, 123
factor deficiencies, 33, 119
as fibrin sealant, 33, 52
hemophilia A, 113
massive transfusion, 78
organ transplantation, 79
von Willebrand disease, 111